Yoga, A Manual for Two or More Doubles Yoga

by

Shar Lee, CYI
&
Dawn R. Mahowald, CYI

Pictures by Karen DeMarco

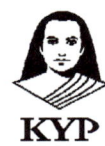

KYP

Kriya Yoga Publications
196 Mountain Rd. P. O. Box 90
Eastman, Quebec, Canada J0E 1P0

Yoga, A Manual for Two or More, Doubles Yoga
By Dawn R. Mahowald, BS, MIM, CYI and Shar Lee, CYI
Photography by: Karen DeMarco

Co-Published in Canada by Kriya Yoga Publications and Unique Yoga, Inc.

Kriya Yoga Publications   Unique Yoga, Inc.
196 Mountain Rd. P. O. Box 90   PO Box 2172
Eastman, Quebec, J0E 1P0   Longmont, CO 80303
Canada   USA
Telephone: (514) 297-0258, or 1-888-252-9642
Fax: 514-297-3957
email: Babaji@generation.net
Website: www.iconn.ca/babaji/

Printed and bound in Canada, First Edition: December, 1997

Cover design and illustration by Mimi Elmore

All the photographs in this book were taken with a digital camera. No film or developing chemicals were used.

Canadian Cataloguing in Publication Data

Lee, Shar 1948-
      Doubles yoga

Includes index.
ISBN 1-895383-08-0

1.   Yoga. I. Mahowald, Dawn R., 1955-
II. De Marco, Karen. III. Title.

RA781.7.L43 1998   613.7'046   C98-900050-8

Consult your physician or health care provider before beginning this or any other exercise program. Neither Unique Yoga, Inc., the authors, models, publisher, printer, distributors, nor sellers of this book assume any responsibility for injuries suffered while practicing these techniques. Do not do these exercise if you are pregnant. If you have any limiting physical, mental, or emotional disorders seek advice from appropriate health care providers about which exercises you should or should not practice.

To all our yoga teachers, past, present, and to come:

NAMASTE

Acknowledgments

Thanks to Karen for the pictures, the fun, and the great excuses for good meals.

Thanks to our husbands and families for encouragement, support, baby-sitting, and dog sitting.

Thanks to Linda Mezger and Phyllis O. Reiche for their much needed and appreciated editing skills.

Thanks to McDougal Photo-Imaging for their help with digital processing.

TABLE OF CONTENTS

TABLE OF CONTENTS, cont.

TABLE OF CONTENTS, cont.

TABLE OF CONTENTS, cont.

TABLE OF CONTENTS, cont.

How to Use this Book

This book is for FUN! A lot technical yoga books are available today. Maybe we'll even write one. They are wonderful. If this is the only yoga book you have, get one or two or more of the serious kind for the yoga you practice by yourself. Then, when you practice yoga alone enjoy all the benefits it offers - stretching, muscle toning and strengthening, and relaxation. Get this book out when you want all the good things yoga has to offer, and you want to LAUGH. Like, when your friends come over, when your kids wants to play, or when your spouse has come home from a hard day at work and wants to unwind - with you. If you're a yoga teacher, take it to class; if you're a yoga student, take it to class. Either way you're in for a different sort of treat; of course, yoga classes are a treat no matter what, aren't they?

To have even more fun with double's yoga, here are some additional ideas and suggestions:

- Check with your health care provider before starting this or any exercise program.

- Contact a qualified yoga teacher if you have any questions.

- Do your yoga in a pleasant environment.

- Wear loose, stretchy, comfortable clothing. There's nothing like a binding waist band to make you feel uncomfortable.

- Practice safely and comfortably; bruises are NOT fun. Try non-slip surfaces such as a wooden floor or an inexpensive "sticky mat" for standing poses and a nice soft carpet or rug for sitting and other poses.

- Don't eat a big meal just before you practice. As with other forms of exercise, you could get indigestion - a great way to spoil your fun. Wait an hour or two after you eat to do yoga.

- Always warm up before doing the major poses. Some people find long, warm showers helpful before they practice.

- Choose a variety of poses during your session, like a few forward bends, a few backward bends, a few standing poses, a couple of inversions, a twist or two, and, of course, a long relaxation at the end. The relaxation poses have always been voted "the most fun" of all of the poses.

- Stick with poses that work for both of you. If you are the more advanced partner, go easy on the other person.

- If you are not as advanced as your partner is, you should set the level of the exercises. If you feel like doing a little more, go ahead and stretch yourself into a new pose. But, stretch yourself with compassion and take care.

- Do each pose only as long as both of you are comfortable in it. Ten breaths is a good number of breaths to stay in a pose.

- Do a workout session of poses only as long as both of you are comfortable. It's not a race or a competition - it's "fun."

Specific Instructions for the Poses

- If each of the Partners is supposed to do something different the instructions will give instructions for each.

- If the Partners are supposed to do the same thing, such as in a mirror image pose, no individual instructions will be given for each Partner.

- If you are unfamiliar with any of the starting positions mentioned, check the "Miscellaneous Poses & Mudras" section in the back of this book.

Have a good time!

WARM UP POSES

Back to Back Breathing (Sukasana)

All Levels

Instructions
1. Start sitting in a mutually agreed upon position on the floor such as straight-legged on a stack of blankets,
2. . . . or in the Cross-Legged Pose (shown),
3. . . . or the Easy Pose*,
4. . . . or the Lotus Pose* and coordinate your breathing by inhaling and exhaling in unison at a pace comfortabe for both Partners.

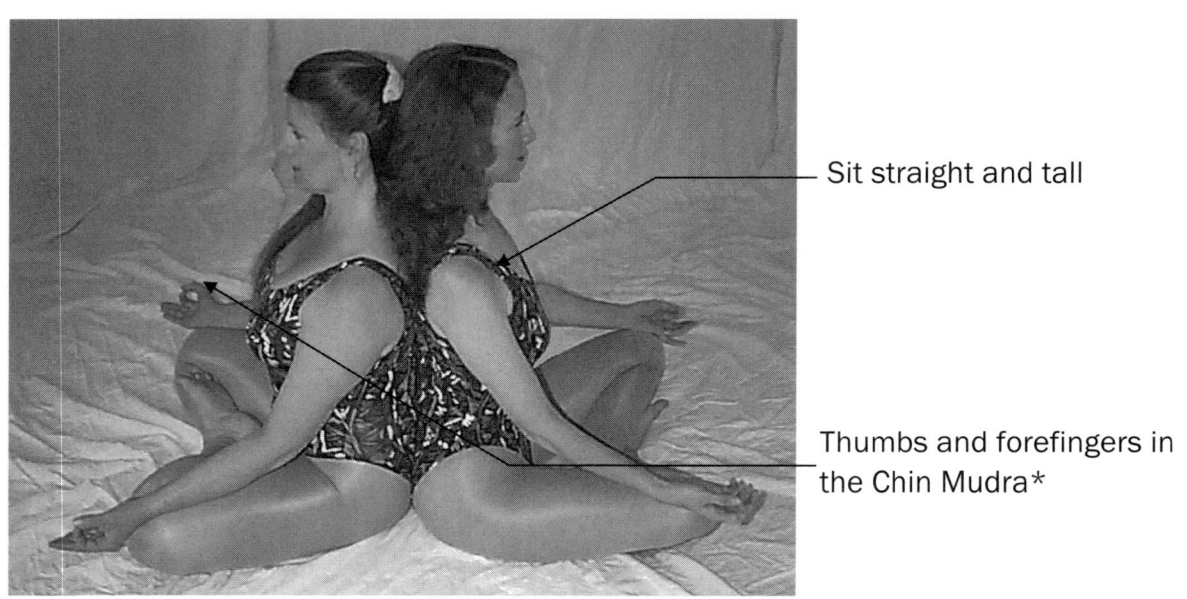

Sit straight and tall

Thumbs and forefingers in the Chin Mudra*

Finding your way in together.

* See Index or Miscellaneous Poses & Mudras section of the Table of Contents to locate pictures of theses poses and finger positions.

Searching (Parivrtta Sukasana 1, Moving)

All Levels

Instructions
1. Start sitting back to back in the Cross-Legged, Easy, or Lotus Pose.
2. EXHALE and twist torso to the RIGHT at the same time.
3. INHALE and twist back to the starting position. Repeat twisting to the LEFT.

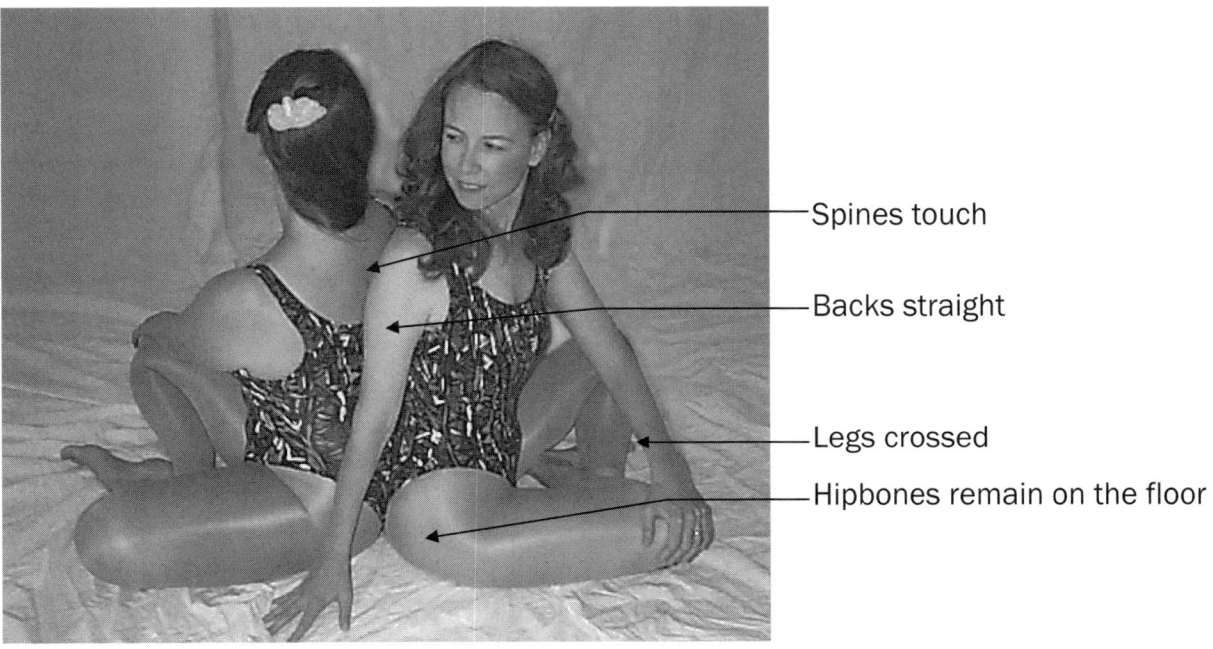

Spines touch

Backs straight

Legs crossed

Hipbones remain on the floor

Where is your Partner, really?

Finding (Parivrtta Sukasana 2, Moving)

All Levels

Instructions
1. Start sitting back to back in the Cross-Legged, Easy, or Lotus Pose.
2. EXHALE and twist torso to Partner 1's RIGHT.
3. INHALE and twist back to the starting position. Repeat twisting to Partner 1 LEFT.

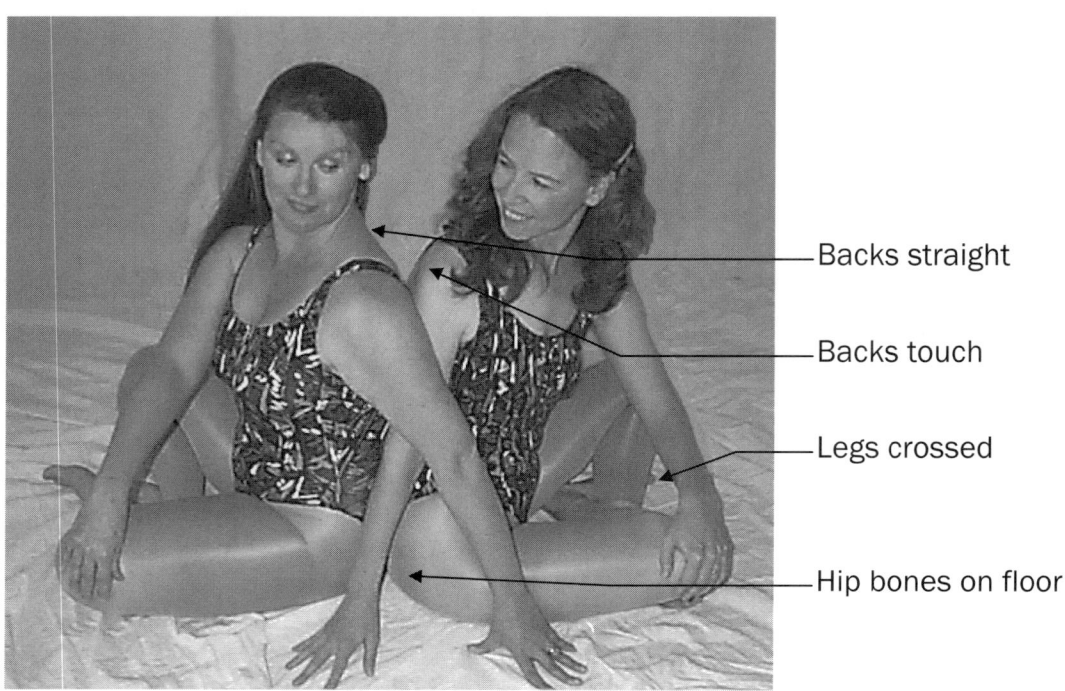

— Backs straight

— Backs touch

— Legs crossed

— Hip bones on floor

Making Contact

Garland (Namaste)

All Levels

Instructions
1. Start sitting back to back with gleuteals and shoulders touching.
2. Partner 1 places their hands on their hips.
3. Partner 2 reaches back with their arms and puts their arms through the "hole made by Partner 1's body and arms.
4. With Partner 2's hands in the "Namaste" or "Prayer" position, both partners pull gently with their arms. Repeat with Partners' arms reversed.

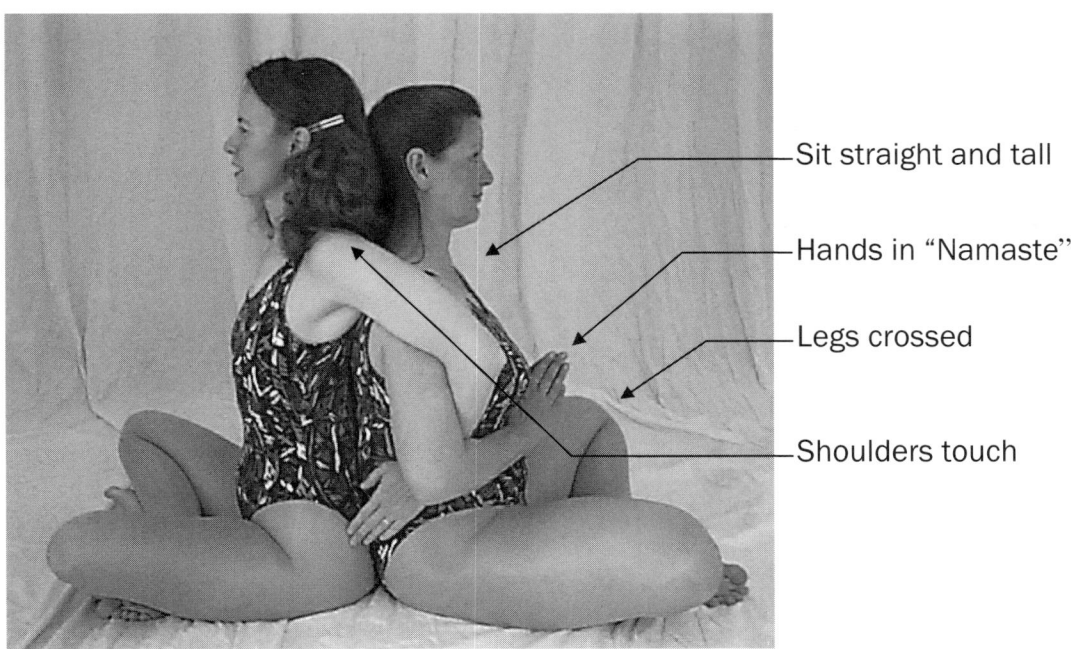

Sit straight and tall

Hands in "Namaste"

Legs crossed

Shoulders touch

Namaste
I honor the place in you where the entire universe resides.
I honor the place in you of love, of light, of truth, of peace.
I honor the place within you where if you are in that place in you and I am in that place in me, there is only one of us.

Cleaning the Mirrors

All Levels

Instructions

1. Start standing face to face with hands palm to palm, but not touching.
2. Starting with Partner 1 as the leader, move together to "clean the mirror" from side to side, . . .
3. top to bottom, and back again to the starting position.
4. After 1-2 minutes let Partner 2 be the leader and repeat.

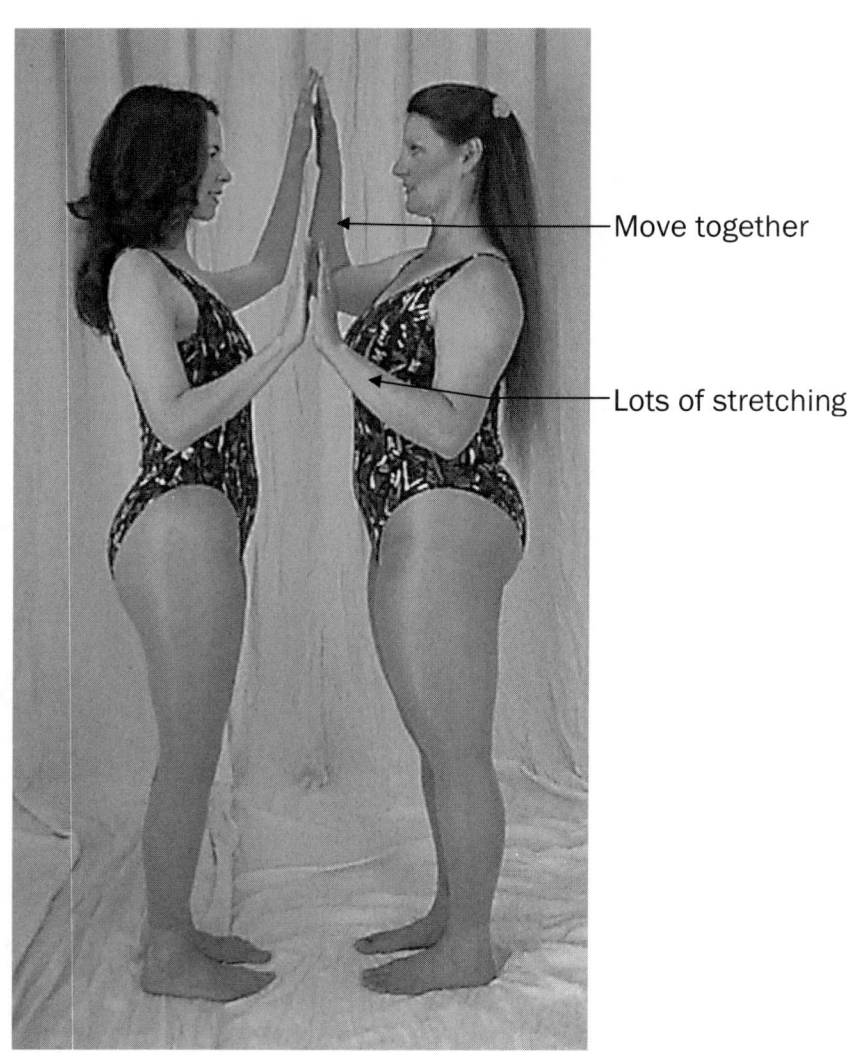

Move together

Lots of stretching

Seeing Yourself in the Mirror

Leg Stretch (Antanasana)

All Levels

Cautions - Do **NOT** pull your Partner's legs any farther than is comfortable.
         - When you are pulling on your Partner's leg, keep your knees bent.

Instructions

1. Start with Partner 1 lying on their side on the floor and Partner 2 standing, straddling Partner 1's legs at mid-thigh (or lower for less flexible Partners).
2. Partner 1 lifts their top leg straight up as high as they comfortably can.
3. Partner 2 firmly grasps Partner 1's leg around the ankle and Partners begin coordination their breathing, inhaling and exhaling in unison.
4. As the Partners EXHALE, Partner 2 gently pulls Partner 1's leg straight out, away from the hip socket.
5. As the Partners INHALE, Partner 2 continues to pull on Partner 1's leg and at the same time bends it at the hip joint and stretches it upward. The Partners continue this way until Partner 1's leg is lifted as high as is comfortable or until Partner 1's lower hip lifts off the floor.

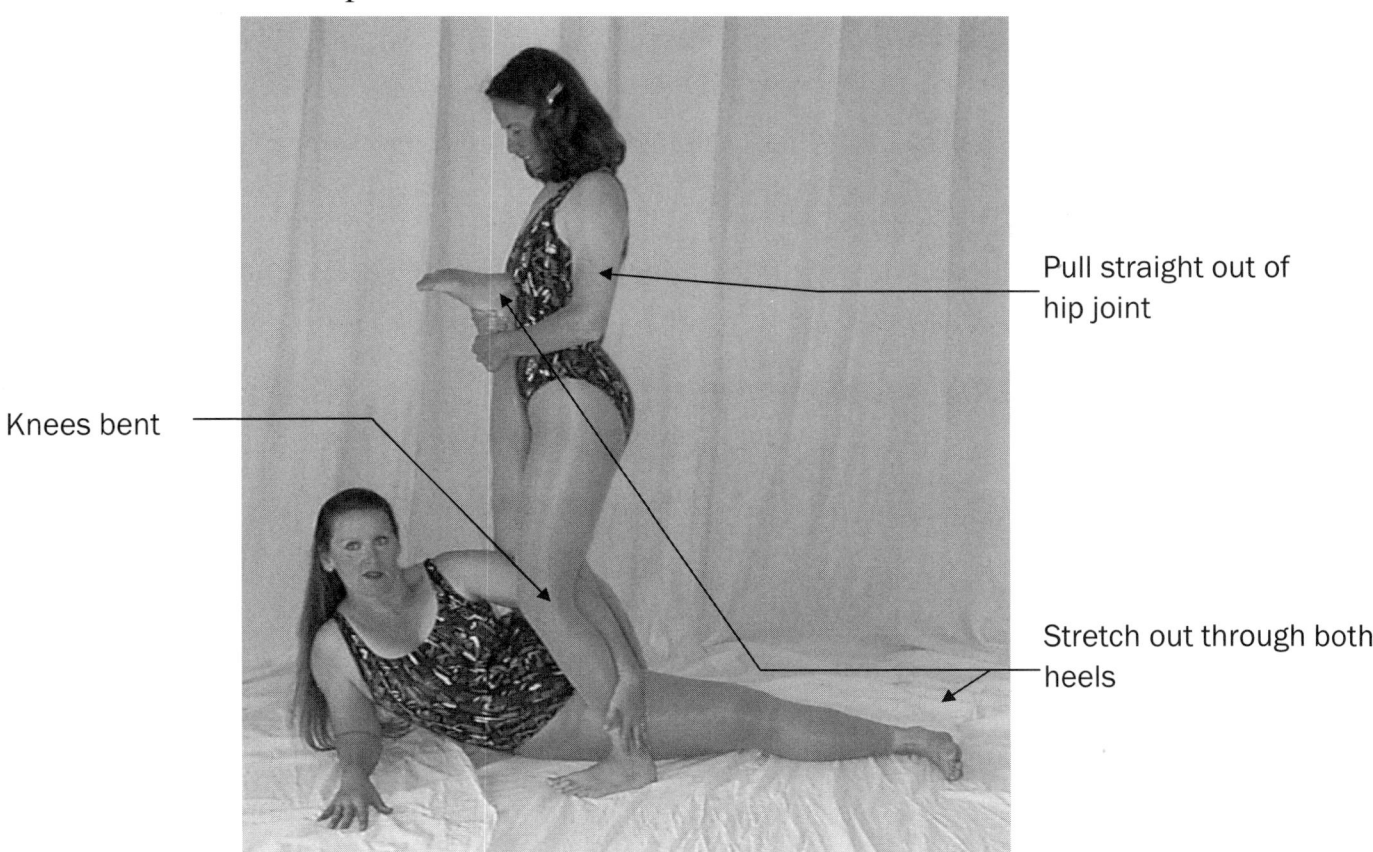

Pull straight out of hip joint

Knees bent

Stretch out through both heels

Another Dance with the Breath

See Saw 1 (Upavistha Konasana, Moving 1)

All Levels

Caution - Do **NOT** pull yourself or your Partner any farther than is comfortable for both of your backs.

Instructions
1. Start sitting face to face, legs spread as wide as is comfortable for each partner with legs bent at the knees. The LESS flexible partner should place their feet on the inside edges of the MORE flexible Partner's legs.

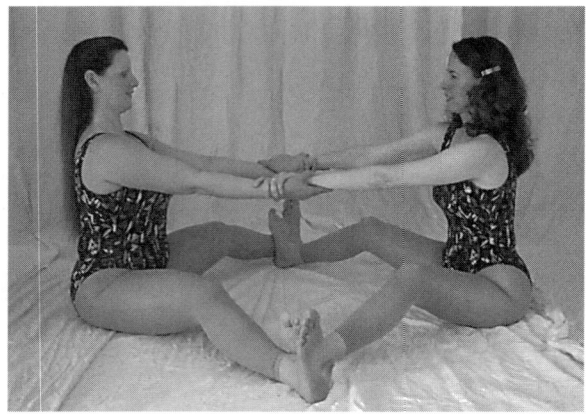

2. Both Partners grasp each other's hands and reverse coordinate their breathing.
3. Partner 1 EXHALES and leans forward as far as they can while Partner 2 INHALES and sits up as far as they can.
4. Then both Partners reverse the movement. Repeat gently and carefully for a total of 10 breaths.

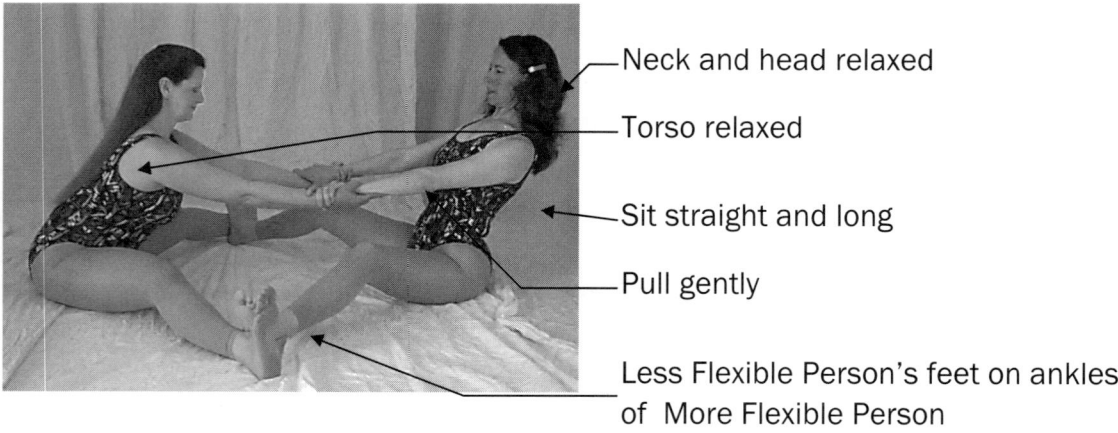

Neck and head relaxed

Torso relaxed

Sit straight and long

Pull gently

Less Flexible Person's feet on ankles of More Flexible Person

Giving One Another Enough Space

Cow - Part 1 (Gomukhasana - Part 1)

All Levels

Instructions

1. Start with Partner 1 sitting on the floor with their LEFT leg crossed over their RIGHT leg as shown and Partner 2 kneeling behind Partner 1 facing their back.
2. Partner 1 raises their RIGHT arm over their head, bends it at the elbow and places their palm on the back of their shoulder blade.
3. Partner 2 places their RIGHT palm on Partner 1's back just below Partner 1's hand.
4. Partner 2 places their LEFT hand on Partner 1's RIGHT elbow and VERY GENTLY pulls back a LITTLE on Partner 1's elbow.

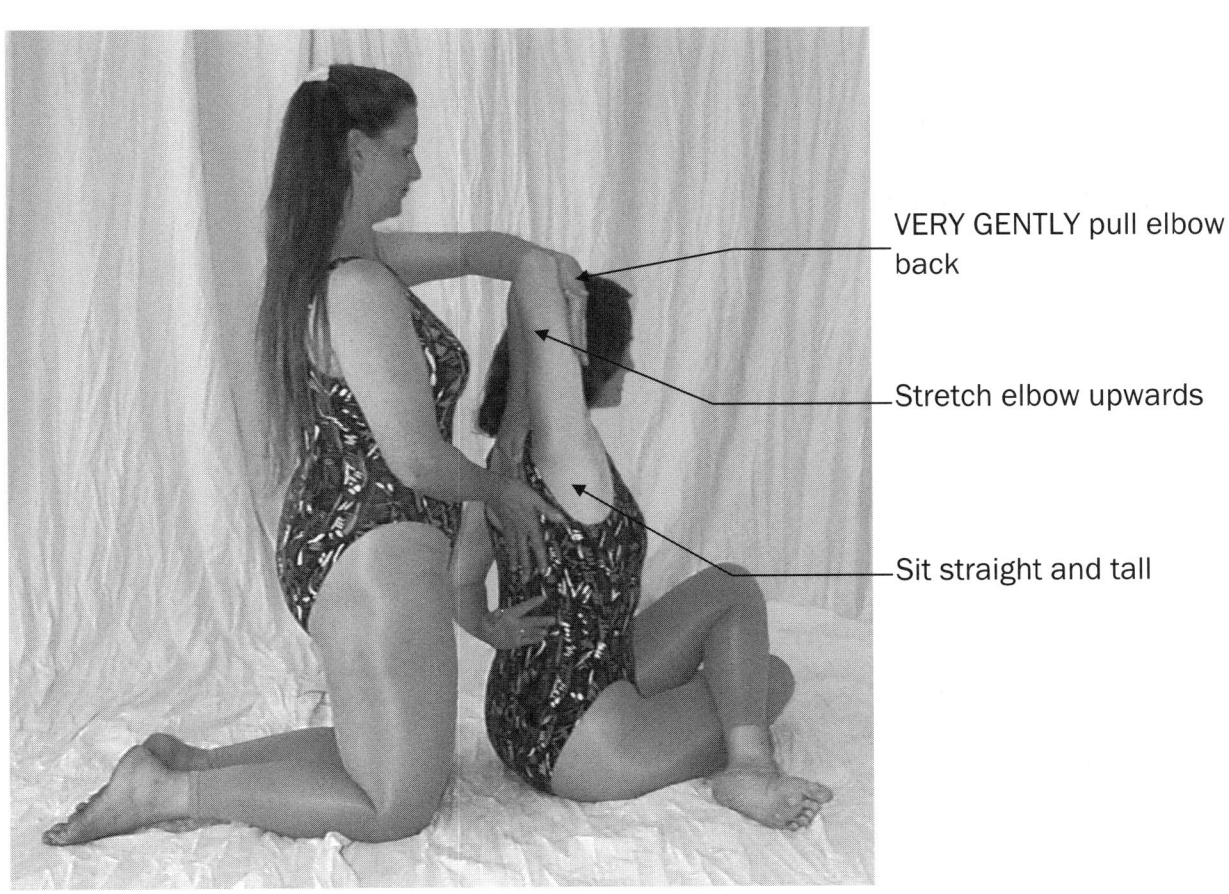

VERY GENTLY pull elbow back

Stretch elbow upwards

Sit straight and tall

Learning How Much You Give and Take

Cow - Part 2 (Gomukhasana - Part 2)

All Levels

Instructions
1. Start with Partner 1 sitting on the floor with their LEFT leg crossed over their RIGHT leg as shown and Partner 2 kneeling behind Partner 1 facing their back.
2. Partner 1 bends their RIGHT arm at the elbow and places their knuckles on the back of their spine. Then they stretch their LEFT arm over their head, bend it at the elbow, and place their palm on the back of their head or neck.
3. Partner 2 places their RIGHT palm on the back of Partner 1's shoulder.
4. Partner 2 grasps Partner 1's LEFT elbow and VERY GENTLY pulls it back SLIGHTLY while holding their RIGHT shoulder steady.

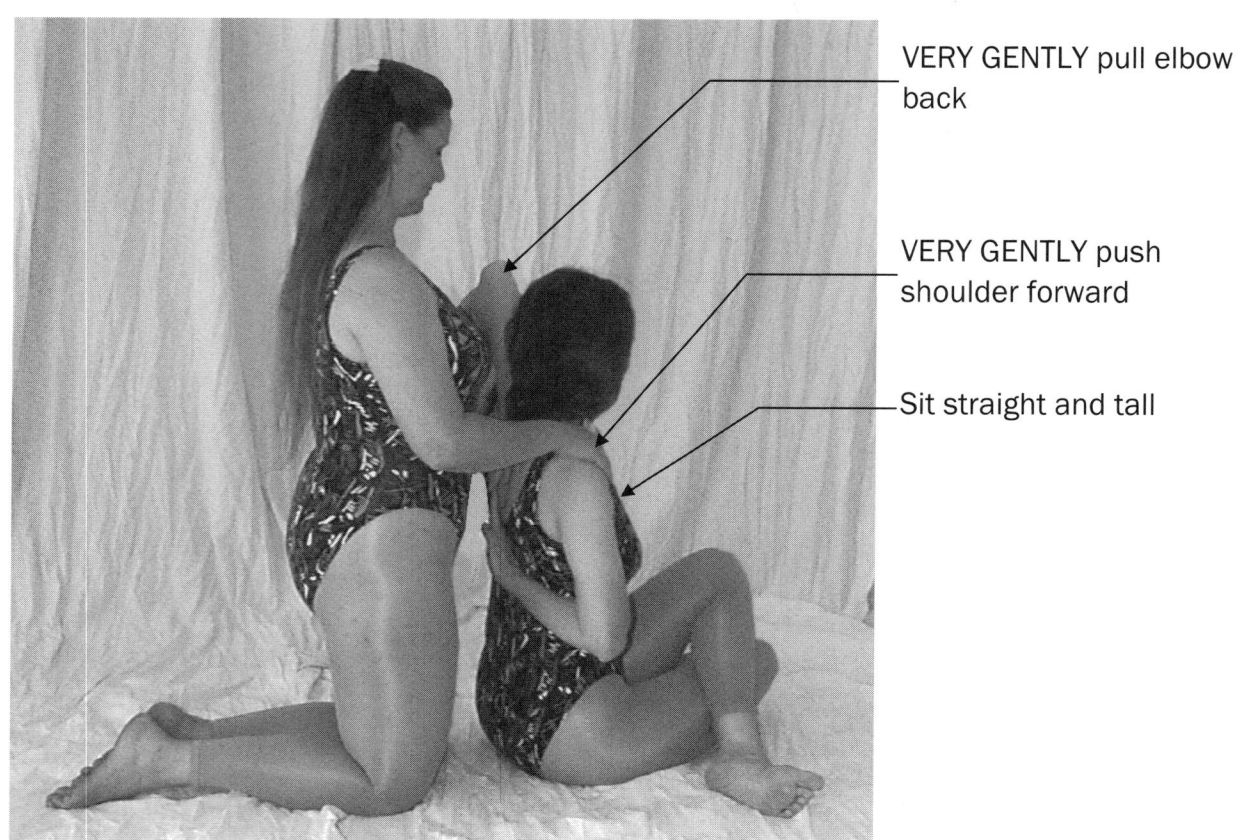

VERY GENTLY pull elbow back

VERY GENTLY push shoulder forward

Sit straight and tall

More Give and Take

Cow - Part 3 (Gomukhasana - Part 3)

All Levels

Instructions

1. Start with Partner 1 sitting on the floor with their LEFT leg crossed over their RIGHT leg as shown and Partner 2 kneeling behind Partner 1 facing their back.
2. Partner 1 bends their LEFT arm at the elbow and places their knuckles on the back of their spine. Then they stretch their RIGHT arm over their head, bend it at the elbow, and place their palm on the back of their head or neck.
3. Partner 2 places a belt in Partner 1's hands.
4. Partner 2 VERY GENTLY pulls back SLIGHTLY on the belt.

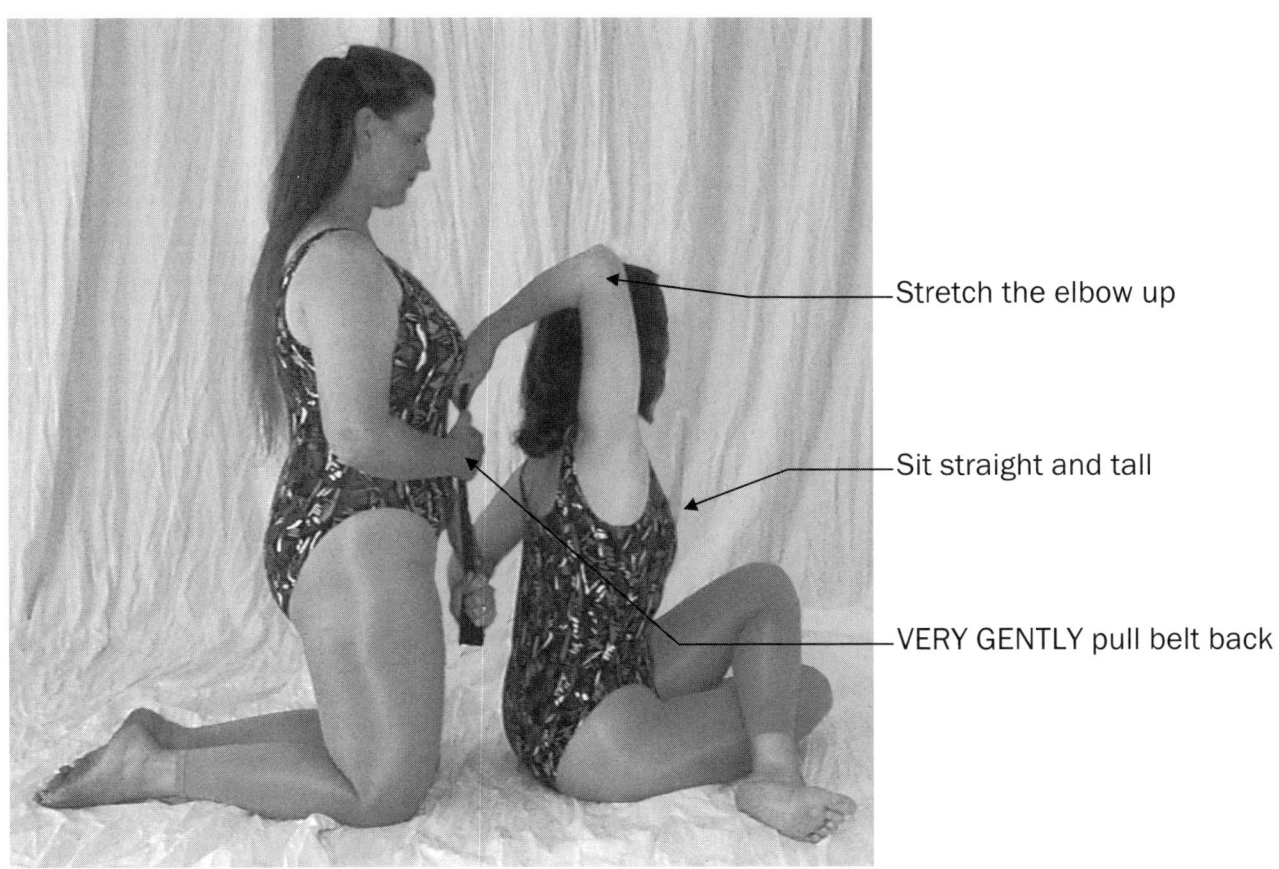

Stretch the elbow up

Sit straight and tall

VERY GENTLY pull belt back

Reaching the Edge of Give and Take

STANDING POSES

Tree Pose (Vrksasana)

All Levels

Instructions
1. Start standing side by side hips 1-2 inches apart.
2. Both Partners bend their OUTSIDE legs at the knees, place the soles of their outside feet on the inside of their thighs just above their knees as shown (you may need to use your hands to assist), and let inside hips touch.
3. Intertwine inside arms so palms touch as shown.
4. Stretch outside arms up and towards center to let palms touch.

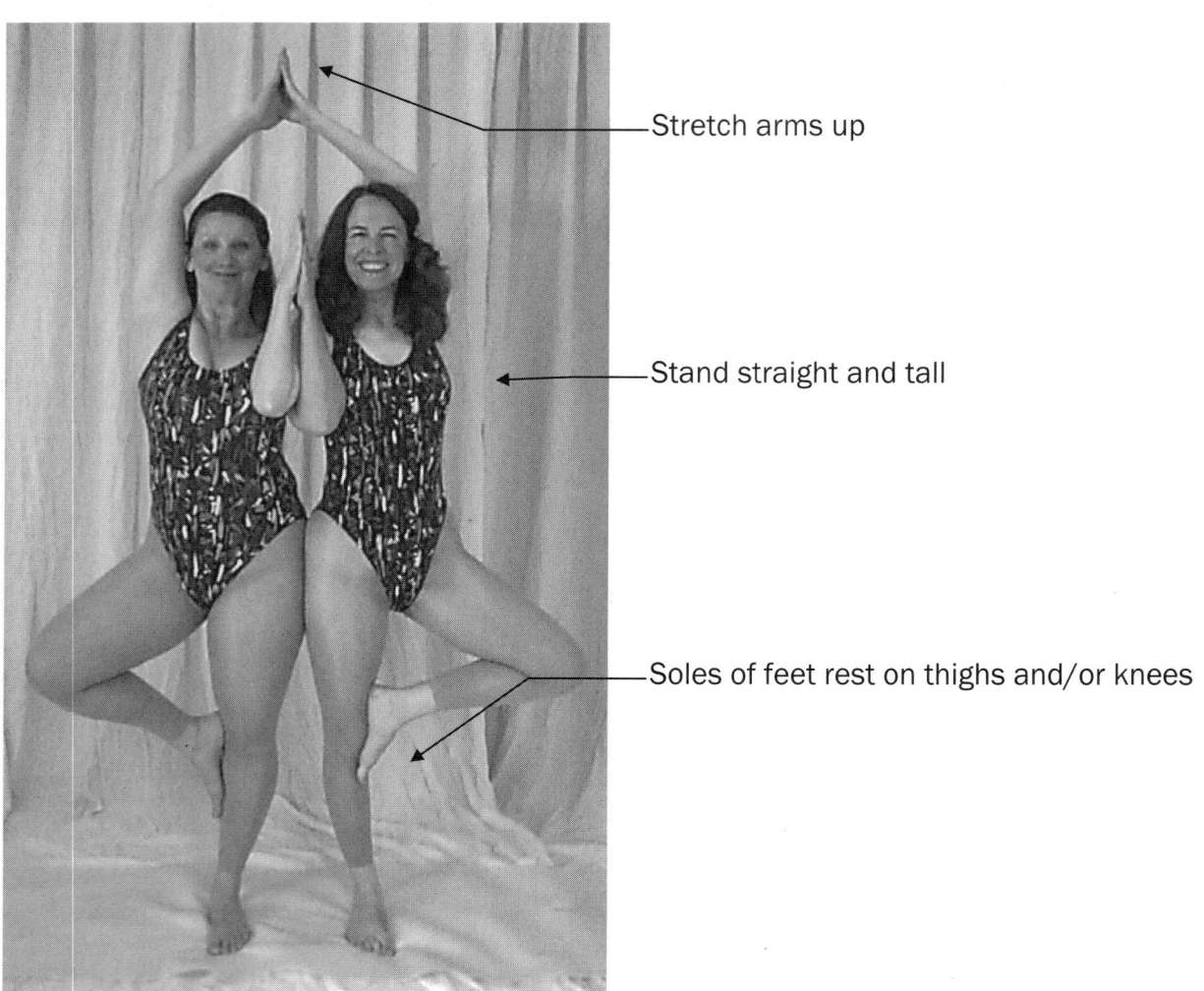

Stretch arms up

Stand straight and tall

Soles of feet rest on thighs and/or knees

Friendship - Roots that Intertwine

Tweedle Dee & Tweedle Dum (Utthita Hasta Padangusthasana 1)

All Levels

Cautions - If you feel you are going to fall, do NOT grab your partner or hold on to them to keep from falling!
- If you feel your Partner is going to fall, LET them fall and catch themselves without interference!

Instructions

1. Start standing side by side facing the same direction and determine which Partner is more flexible in the hips and legs.
2. Step apart until each Partners' palm can rest, straight armed on the other Partners' shoulder.
3. The LESS FLEXIBLE Partner raises their inside leg IN FRONT of the MORE FLEXIBLE Partner and places their foot in the MORE FLEXIBLE Partner's OUTSIDE hand.
4. The MORE FLEXIBLE Partner raises their INSIDE leg BEHIND the LESS FLEXIBLE Partner and places their foot in the LESS FLEXIBLE Partner's OUTSIDE hand.

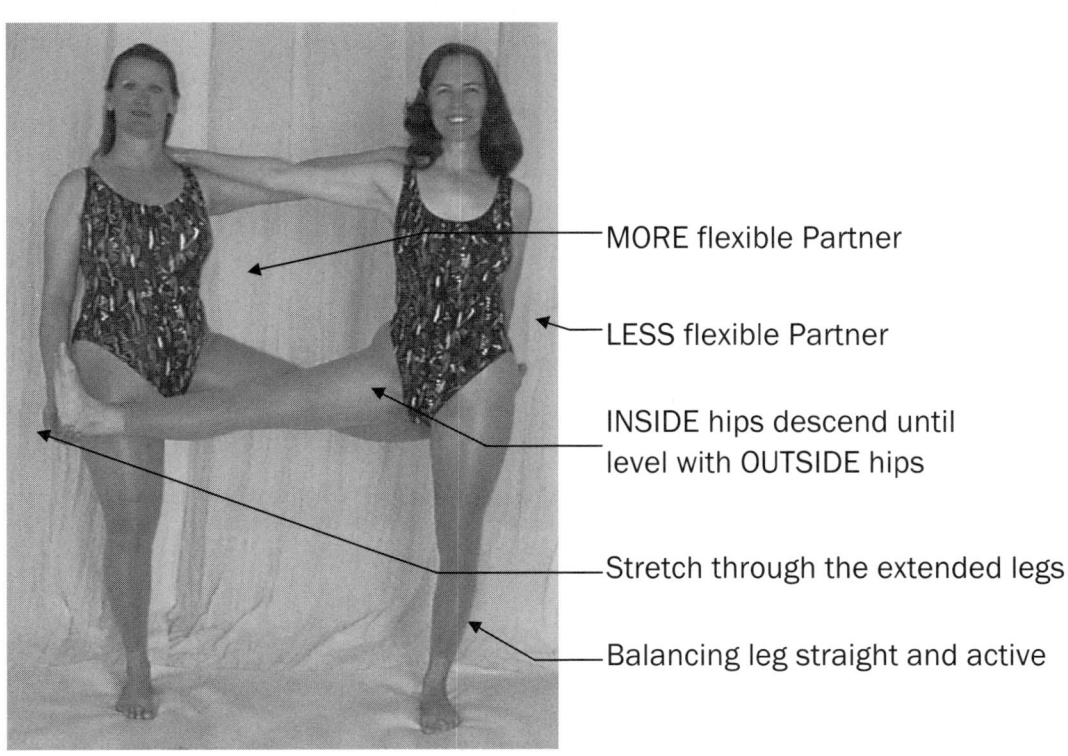

MORE flexible Partner

LESS flexible Partner

INSIDE hips descend until level with OUTSIDE hips

Stretch through the extended legs

Balancing leg straight and active

Do Ujjayi Breath in Unison.

Eye Gaze (Utthita Hasta Padangusthasana 2)

All Levels

Cautions - If you feel your Partner is going to fall, LET them fall and catch themselves without interference!
- If you feel you are going to fall, do NOT grab your partner or hold on to them to keep from falling!

Instructions
1. Start standing face to face far enough apart that the SHORTER Partner's finger tips can touch the TALLER Partner's chest.
2. Partner 1 places their LEFT heel in Partner 2's RIGHT hand.
3. Partner 2 does the same.
4. Partners touch LEFT hands palm to palm and extend arms upwards.

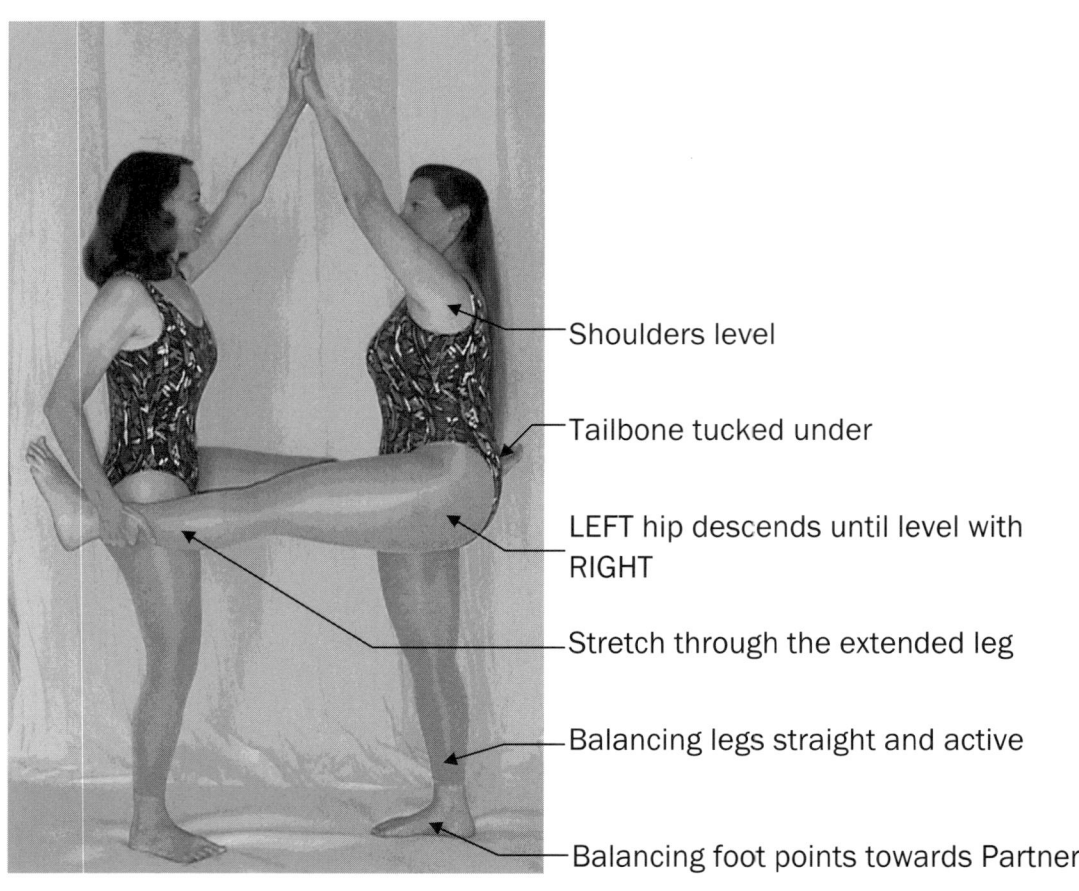

- Shoulders level
- Tailbone tucked under
- LEFT hip descends until level with RIGHT
- Stretch through the extended leg
- Balancing legs straight and active
- Balancing foot points towards Partner

Support - Feel the strength in your standing leg and how it roots down into the floor. Then make eye contact and feel how your Partner is supporting your lifted leg.

Turning the Other Cheek (Utthita Hasta Padangusthasana 3)

All Levels

Cautions - If you feel you are going to fall, do NOT grab your partner or hold on to them to keep from falling!
- If you feel your Partner is going to fall, LET them fall and catch themselves without interference.

Instructions
1. Start standing face to face far enough apart so the SHORTER Partner's hands touch the side of the TALLER Partner's waist. Partners' LEFT arms should be wrapped behind their backs and LEFT hands reaching out towards the RIGHT.
2. Partner 1 raises their LEFT leg, places their LEFT heel in Partner 2's LEFT hand and then places their RIGHT hand on Partner 1's RIGHT shoulder.
3. Partner 2 does the same.
4. Make eye contact with your Partner when you have both placed your legs in your Partner's hand. Twist torsos to the LEFT. As you twist move your gaze as your body turns.

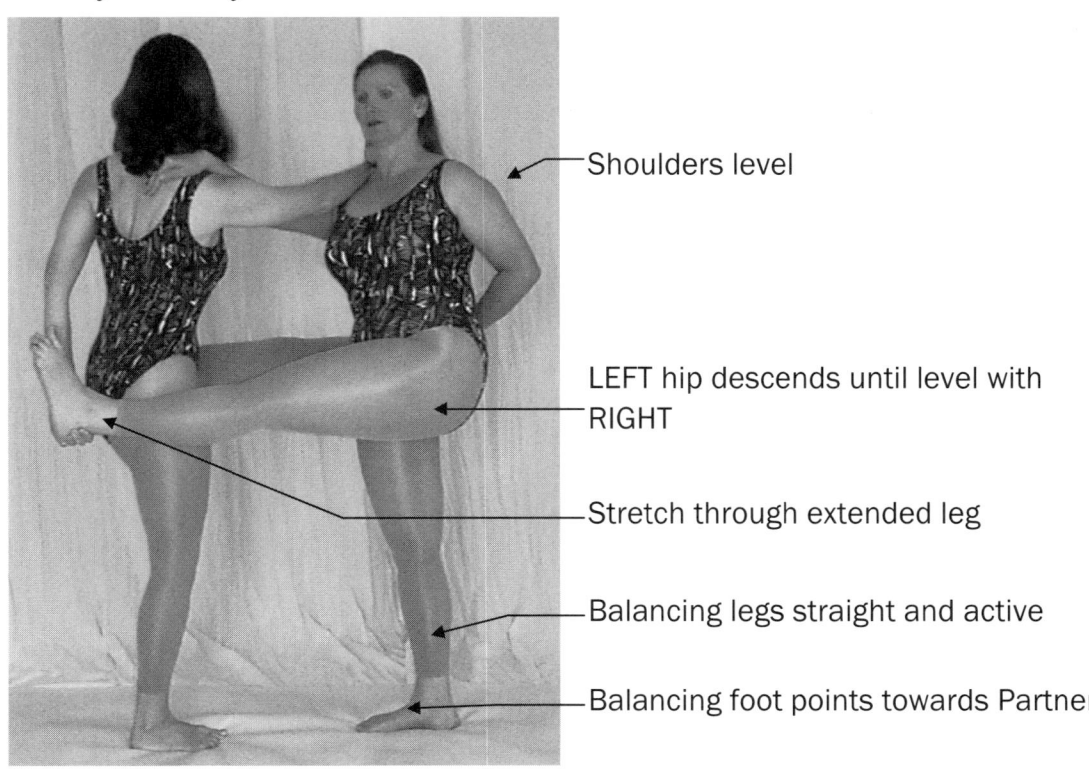

Shoulders level

LEFT hip descends until level with RIGHT

Stretch through extended leg

Balancing legs straight and active

Balancing foot points towards Partner

Tartak

Celtic Braid (Utthita Hasta Padangusthasana 4)

Intermediate/Advanced Levels

Cautions - If you feel you are going to fall, do NOT grab your partner or hold on to them to keep from falling!
   - If you feel your Partner is going to fall, LET them fall and catch themselves without interference.

Instructions
1. Start standing face to face far enough apart that the SHORTER Partner's palms can rest on the TALLER Partner's shoulder.
2. Partner 1 raises their LEFT leg and places their LEFT heel on Partner 2's RIGHT shoulder.
3. Partner 2 does the same.
4. Partners place their hands on the other Partner's shoulders.

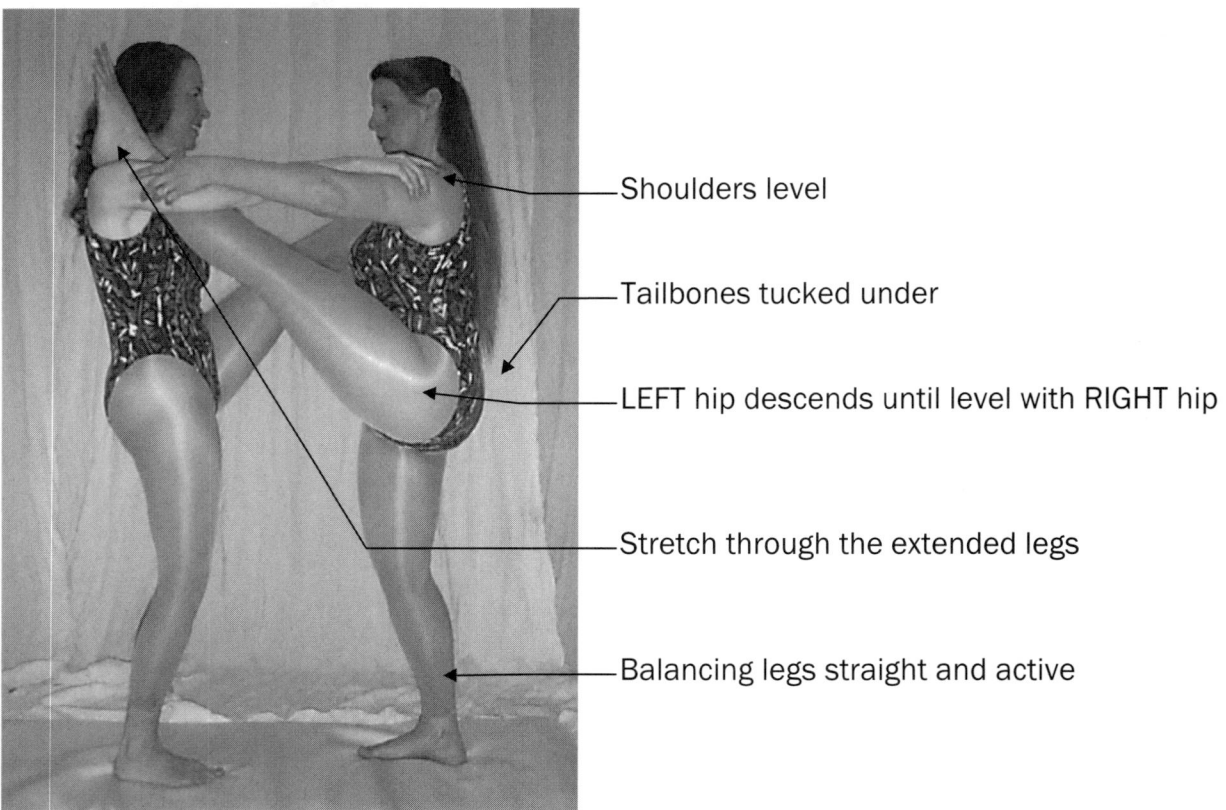

Shoulders level

Tailbones tucked under

LEFT hip descends until level with RIGHT hip

Stretch through the extended legs

Balancing legs straight and active

Ascension - Shouldering Each Others Joy

Twisting Triangle (Parivrtta Trikonasana)

All Levels

Instructions

1. Start standing face to face 8 - 12" inches apart.
2. Partner 1 steps their foot out 2 1/2 - 3' out to their RIGHT, turns it 90 degrees away from midline, turns the other foot 45 degrees towards midline, and rotates their torso to their RIGHT. Partner 2 does these same, but goes to their LEFT so both are facing the same direction.
3. Both Partners bend forward from the hips, twist their torsos outwards, and stretch their arms out from their sides.
4. Partners' lower arms should cross and their upper hands should clasp. Repeat on the other side

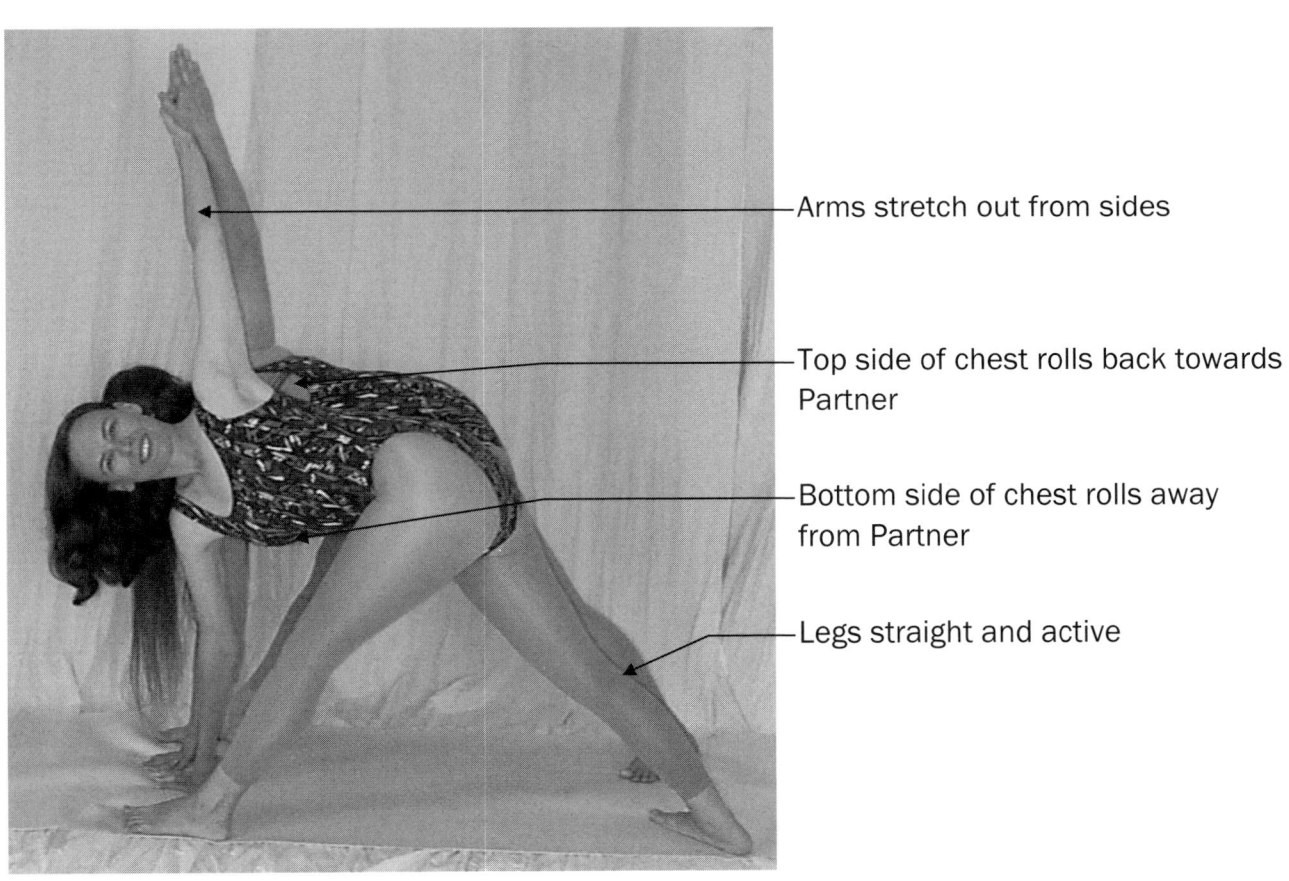

Arms stretch out from sides

Top side of chest rolls back towards Partner

Bottom side of chest rolls away from Partner

Legs straight and active

A Gateway to Open the Heart.

Sunrise (Virbhadrasana I)

All Levels

Instructions

1. Start standing side to side facing opposite directions with the OUTSIDE legs spread out two to three feet (the exact distance depends on height of each Partner).
2. Turn OUTSIDE feet 90 degrees to the OUTSIDE, turn INSIDE foot 45 degrees towards the OUTSIDE with the INSIDE feet touching along the "little toe" edge, and turn upper body to face the OUTSIDE.
3. Raise both arms over heads, bend OUTSIDE/FRONT legs at the knees until lower legs are perpendicular to the floor, tilt heads back until gazes rest on the ceiling.
4. Reach back and interlace fingers with Partner. Imagine you and your partner lifting the sun up into the sky with the tips of your fingers.

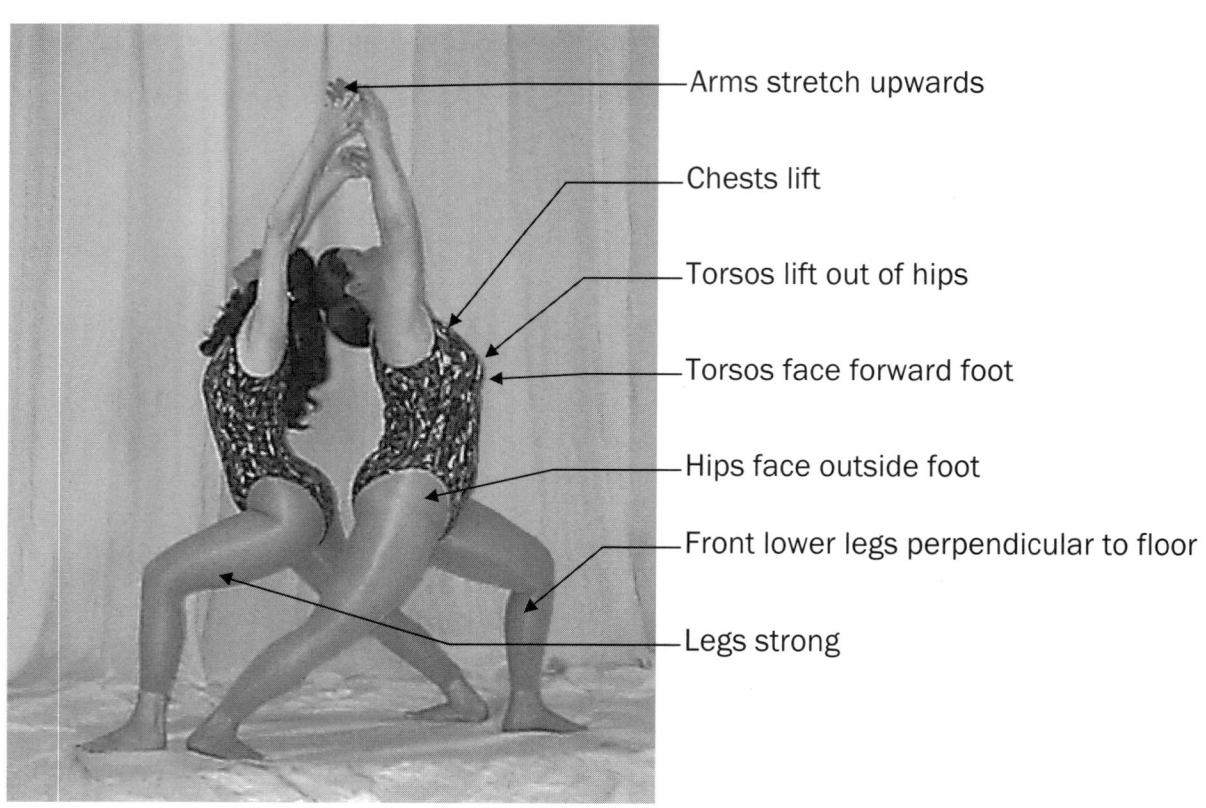

Arms stretch upwards

Chests lift

Torsos lift out of hips

Torsos face forward foot

Hips face outside foot

Front lower legs perpendicular to floor

Legs strong

Energy Rising

Loveseat (Virbhadrasana II - 1)

All Levels

Instructions

1. Start standing side by side, facing the opposite direction, with INSIDE legs and edges of feet touching and OUTSIDE legs spread out 3 - 4 1/2 feet (the exact distance depends on height of each Partner).
2. Stretch OUTSIDE arms straight out to the side, and grasp one another's INSIDE forearms at the elbow.
3. Turn OUTSIDE feet 90 degrees to the OUTSIDE, turn INSIDE feet 45 degrees towards the OUTSIDE with INSIDE edges of feet still touching. Make eye contact for one or two breaths, then EXHALE and turn heads towards the OUTSIDE arms.
4. Bend OUTSIDE legs at the knees until lower legs are perpendicular to the floor and slide the INSIDE hands down one another's arms until each Partner is gripping the other's wrist.

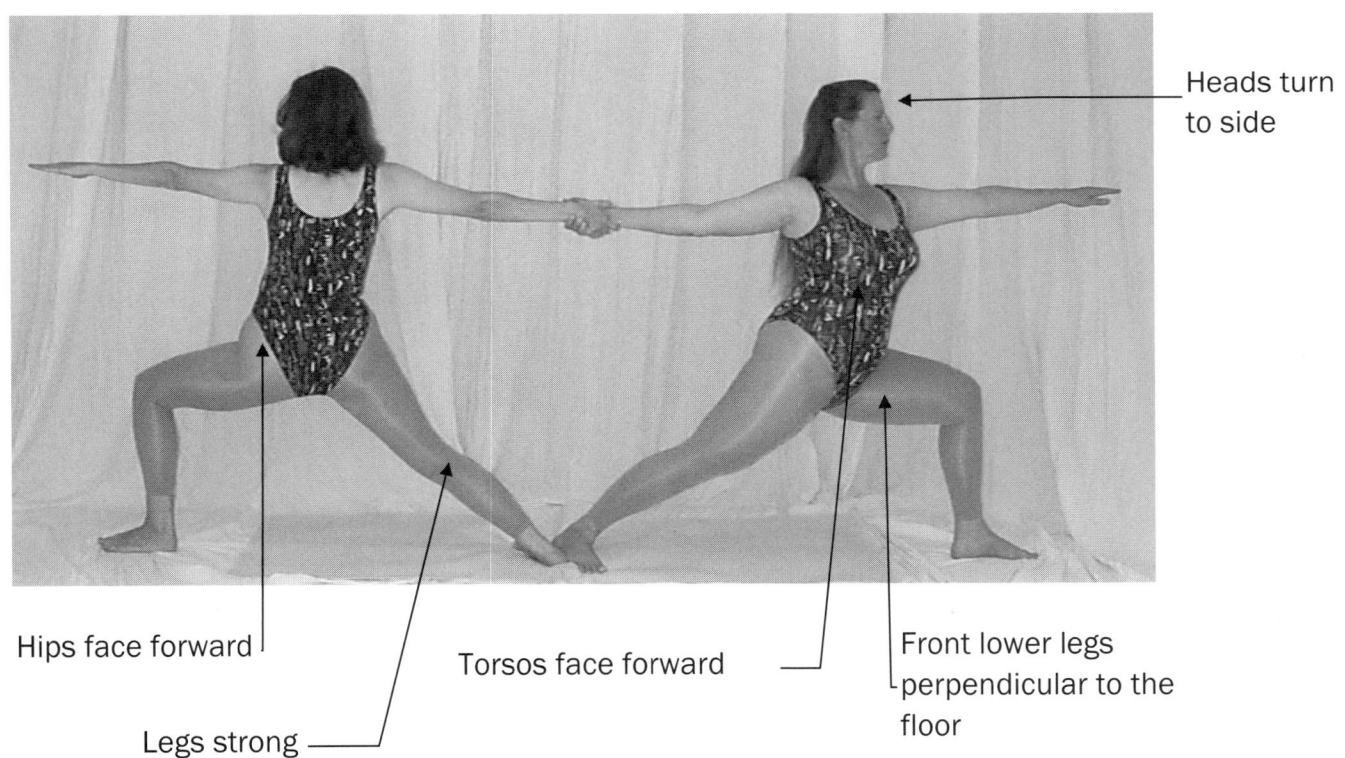

Heads turn to side

Hips face forward

Torsos face forward

Legs strong

Front lower legs perpendicular to the floor

Looking In & Looking Away

The Warrior Pose II (Virbhadrasana II - 2)

All Levels

Instructions
1. Start standing back to back, with hips and shoulders touching.
2. Partner 1 steps their RIGHT foot out 2 1/2 - 3' out to their RIGHT, turns it 90 degrees away from midline, and turns the other foot 45 degrees towards midline. Partner 2 does these same, but starts with their LEFT foot so the Partners are mirror images of one another.
3. Partner 1 bends their RIGHT leg at the knee until the lower leg is perpendicular to the floor. At the same time Partner 2 does the same with their LEFT leg. Torsos remain facing forward.
4. Stretch arms straight out to the side, let hands and arms touch, and turn heads towards bent leg. Repeat on the other side.

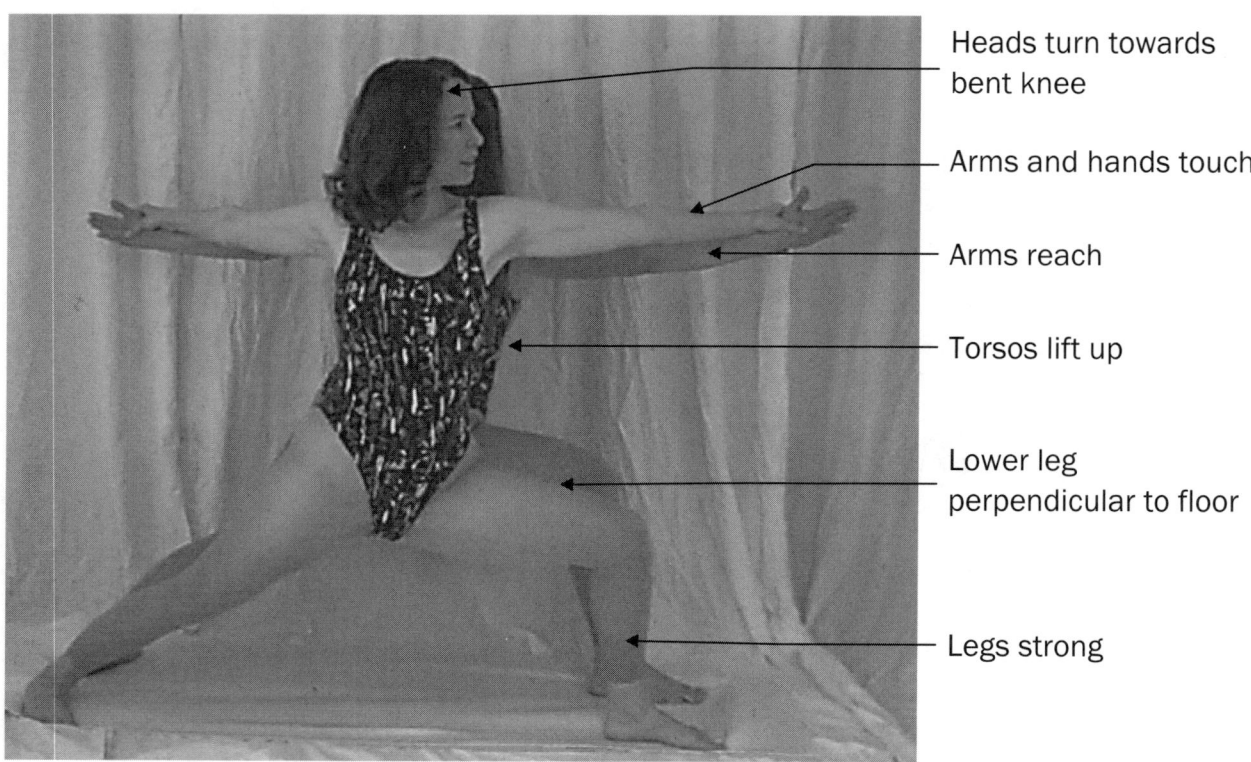

Heads turn towards bent knee

Arms and hands touch

Arms reach

Torsos lift up

Lower leg perpendicular to floor

Legs strong

On Guard

Pivot (Virbhadrasana III)

Intermediate/Advanced Levels

Cautions - If you feel like you are going to fall, do NOT grab your partner or hold on to them to keep from falling!
- If you feel like your Partner is going to fall, LET them fall and catch themselves without interference.

Instructions
1. Start standing face to face, four to six feet apart (the exact distance depends on height of each Partner).
2. Bow and adjust distance so the crowns of heads just touch.
3. Return to the starting position, INHALE and raise arms up over heads, shift balance to the LEFT legs, and stretch out through RIGHT heels.
4. Pivot at LEFT hip joints until torsos and RIGHT legs are horizontal, and crowns of heads are touching. Then, place hands on Partners' shoulder blades.

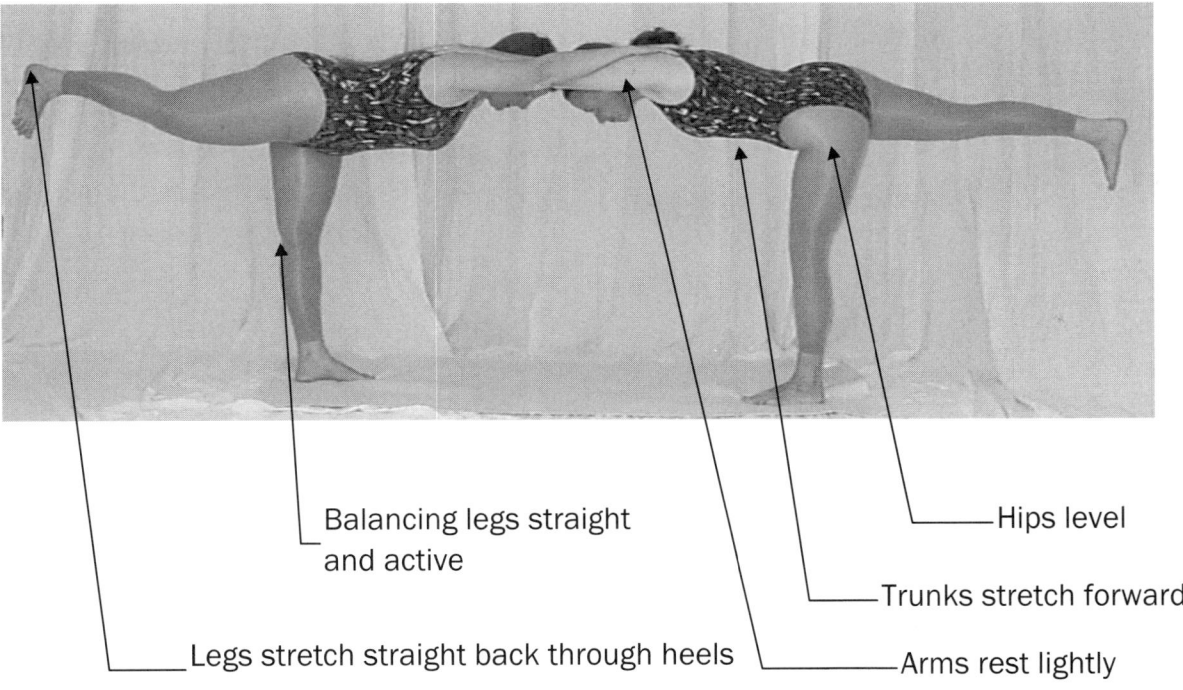

Balancing legs straight and active

Hips level

Trunks stretch forward

Legs stretch straight back through heels

Arms rest lightly

Interconnectedness - Stretch together into each other's past and future and feel the inteconnectedness of life.

The Pinball Pose (Parsvakonasana)

Intermediate/Advanced Levels

Cautions - If you feel like you are going to fall, do NOT grab your partner or hold on to them to keep from falling!
 - If you feel like your Partner is going to fall, LET them fall and catch themselves without interference.

Special Pre-Instructions

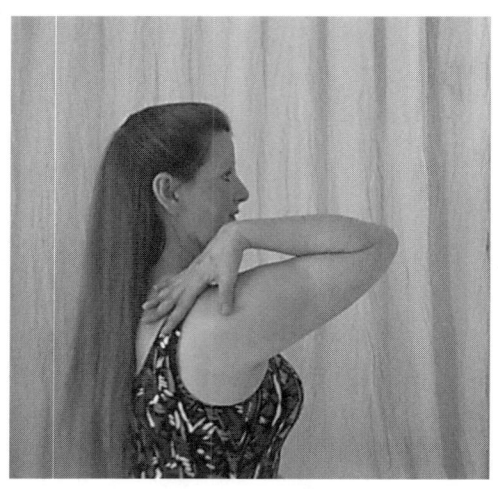

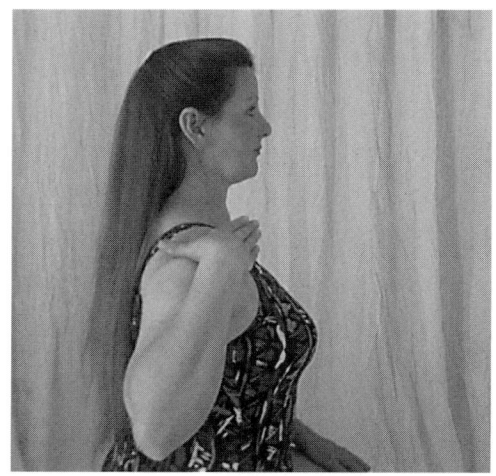

1. Touch RIGHT fingers to shoulder with elbow facing forward and straight out.

2. Swing arm down with the elbow slightly out.

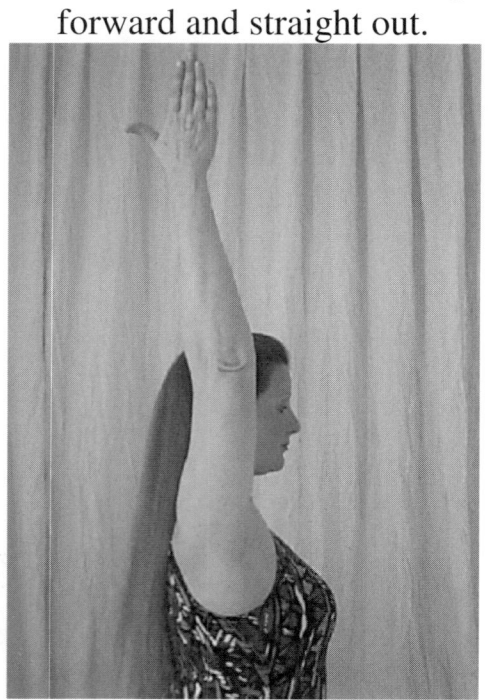

3. Extend arm straight up. This sequence of movements allows the arm to stretch straight up in a very comfortable way. When you stretch your arm in the Pinball Pose, try this series of movements to get the best, most comfortable stretch.

Instructions

1. Start standing back to back, four to six inches apart.
2. Partners step their RIGHT feet out 3-4' to their RIGHT, turn them 90 degrees away from midline, and turn the other feet 45 degrees towards midline.
3. Partners bend their RIGHT legs at the knees until the lower legs are perpendicular to the floor. Torsos remain facing forward.
4. Partners stretch lower arms straight down in back of their bent leg and rest their hands on the floor nest to their feet, and move their arms as shown on the previous page. Partners let hands and arms touch, turn heads towards the fronts of their bodies, and STRETCH. Repeat on the other side.

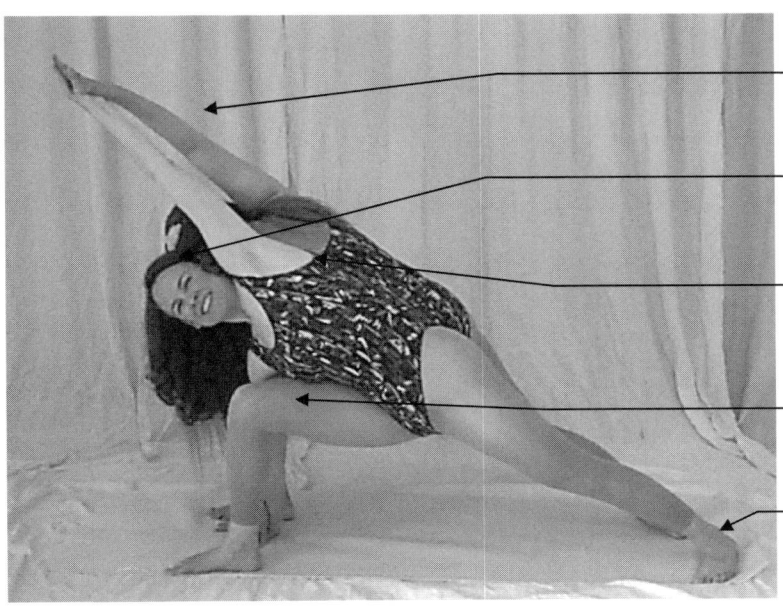

Stretch entire side of body

Heads could also turn to look at extended hands

Top ribs roll back towards Partner and bottom ribs roll away from Partner

Bent leg strong and supportive

Outside edge of foot presses down

Launching Rockets

Split Leg Forward Bend (Parsvotanasana)

All Levels

Instructions

1. Start standing. Partner 1 steps their RIGHT foot out 2 1/2 - 3' to their RIGHT, turns it 90 degrees away from midline, turns the other foot 45 degrees towards midline, and turns torso to the right.
2. Partner 2 does the same. The Partners sitting bones should touch.
3. Partners bend forward from the hips until their torsos rest on their RIGHT legs or as far as is comfortable.
4. Partners move hands into the Namaste hand position* or clasp hands behind their backs. Repeat on the other side.

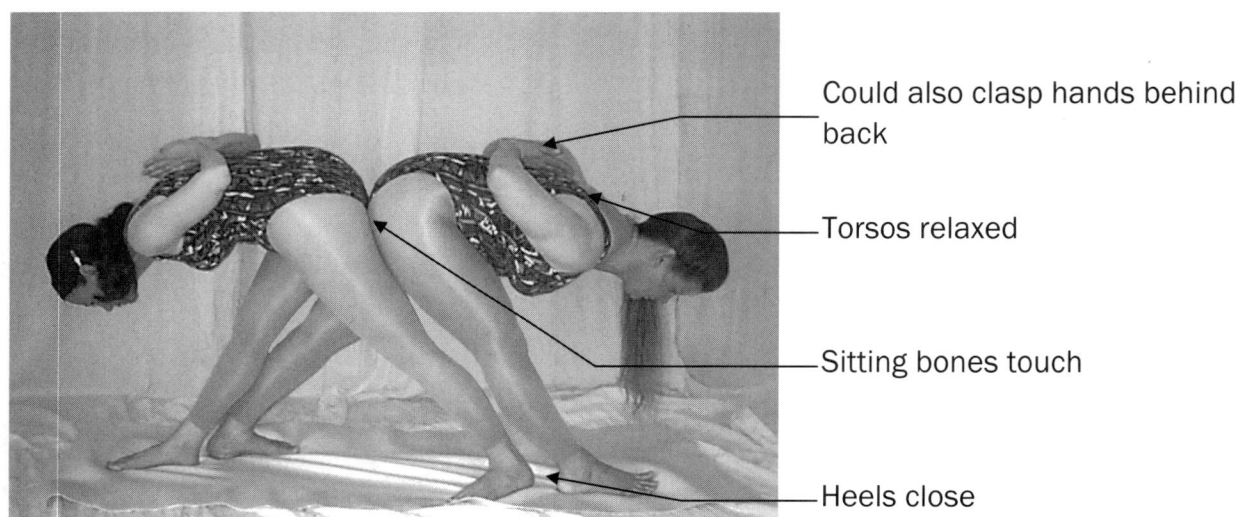

Could also clasp hands behind back

Torsos relaxed

Sitting bones touch

Heels close

Solid Surrender

* See Index or Table of Contents for the Namaste hand position

Double Moon (Ardha Chandrasana 1)

Intermediate Level

Cautions - If you feel you are going to fall, do NOT grab your partner or hold on to them to keep from falling!
- If you feel like your Partner is going to fall, LET them fall and catch themselves without interference.

Instructions
1. Start standing back to back.
2. Partner 1 turns their RIGHT foot 90 degrees to the RIGHT and Partner 2 turns their LEFT foot 90 degrees to the LEFT.
3. Raise arms straight out from sides, then stretch and bend into pose.
4. Touch heels on the extended legs, turn heads to look up, and intertwine upper and lower arms.

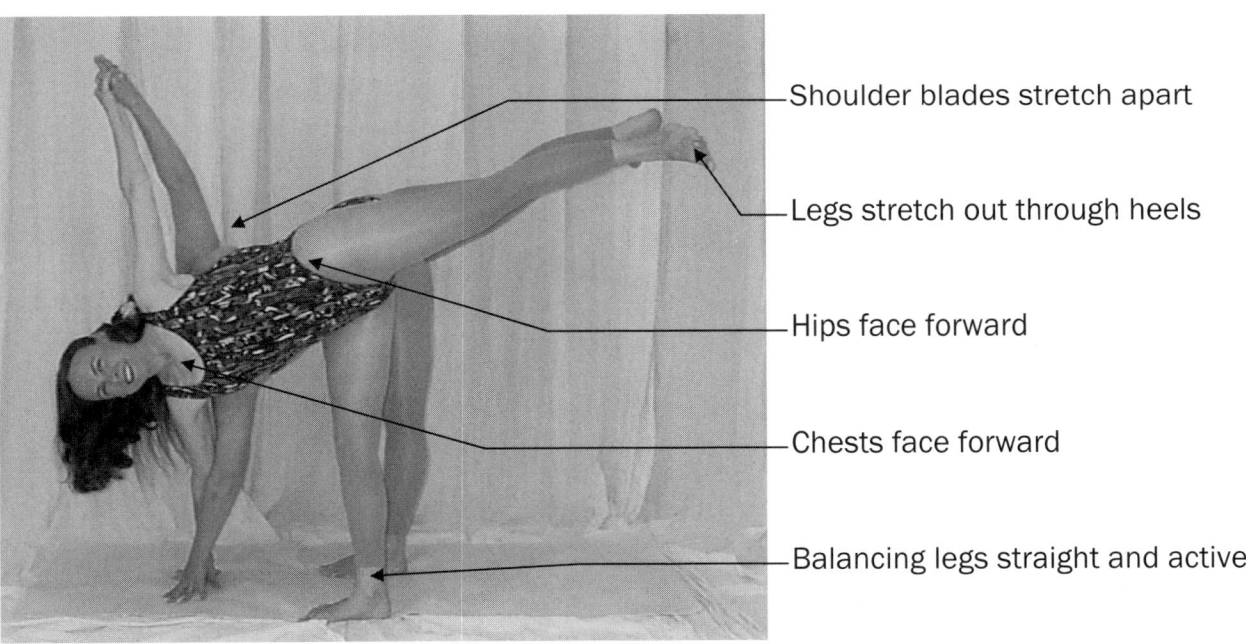

Shoulder blades stretch apart

Legs stretch out through heels

Hips face forward

Chests face forward

Balancing legs straight and active

Learning to Extend - Do you remember how your parent encouraged you to reach out and was always there behind you for support?

Waxing Moon (Ardha Chandrasana 2)

Intermediate Level

Cautions - If you feel you are going to fall, do NOT grab your partner or hold on to them to keep from falling.
- If you feel your Partner is going to fall, LET them fall and catch themselves without interference.
- DO NOT let your leg touch your Partner's head; you could accidentally kick them if you fall.

Instructions
1. Start standing back to back.
2. Both Partners turn LEFT feet 90 degrees towards the LEFT.
3. Raise arms straight out from sides and bend towards the LEFT into the pose.
4. Touch tops of hips and turn heads to look forward.

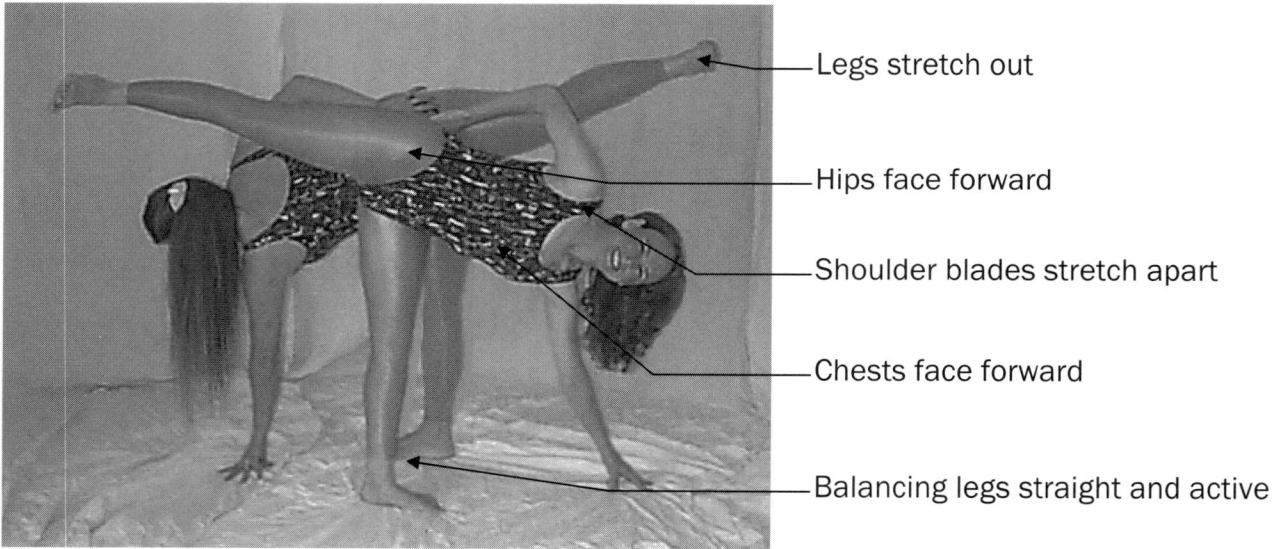

— Legs stretch out

— Hips face forward

— Shoulder blades stretch apart

— Chests face forward

— Balancing legs straight and active

Extending in Opposite Directions - Do you remember how your parent made it possible for you to discover your own individuality?

New Moon (Ardha Chandrasana 3)

Advanced Level

Cautions - If you feel you are going to fall, do NOT grab your partner or hold on to them to keep from falling.
- If you feel your Partner is going to fall, LET them fall and catch themselves without interference.
- DO NOT let your leg touch your Partner's head; you could accidentally kick them if you fall.

Instructions
1. Start standing back to back.
2. Both Partners turn LEFT feet 90 degrees towards the LEFT.
3. Raise arms straight out from sides, bend towards the LEFT into the pose (hips will touch lightly).
4. Lightly grasp Partner's feet as shown and turn heads to look forward.

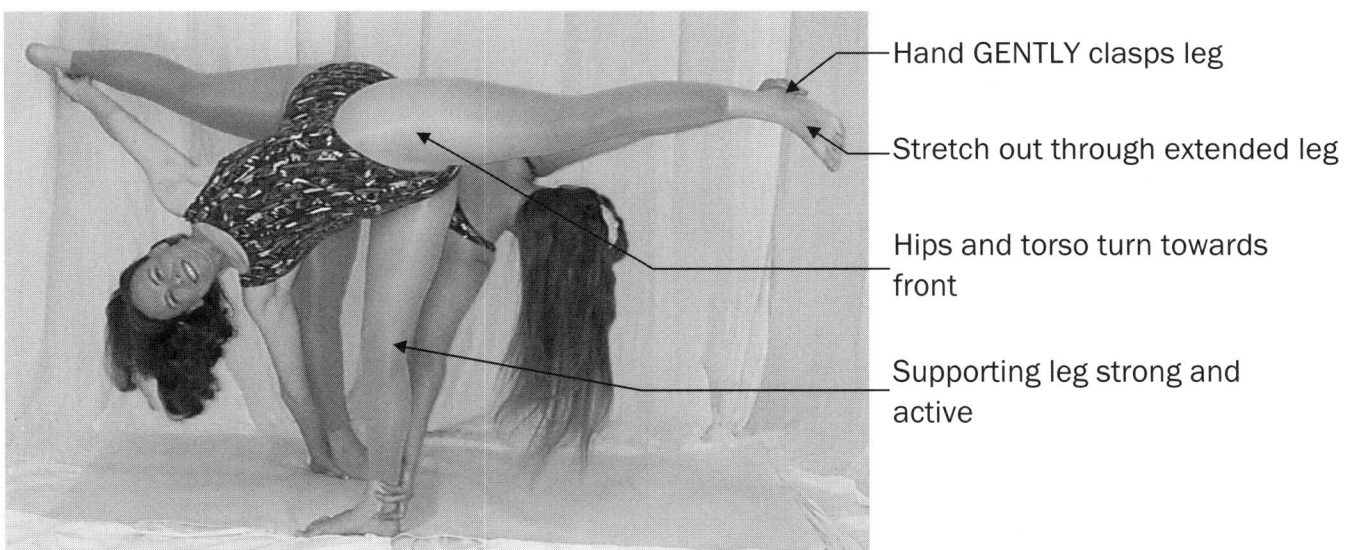

Hand GENTLY clasps leg

Stretch out through extended leg

Hips and torso turn towards front

Supporting leg strong and active

New Moon - Do you remember when you became the parent?

King's Dancer 1 (Natarajasana 1)

Intermediate/Advanced Levels

Cautions - If you feel you are going to fall, do NOT grab your partner or hold on to them to keep from falling!
- If you feel your Partner is going to fall, LET them fall and catch themselves without interference.

Instructions
1. Start standing back to back one to two feet apart (the exact distance will be determined by the flexibility of each Partner's back and shoulders).
2. Bend the LEFT leg at the knee and grasp the front of the ankle with the LEFT hand.
3. Reach up and back with RIGHT arm and hand until you can grasp one another's hands.

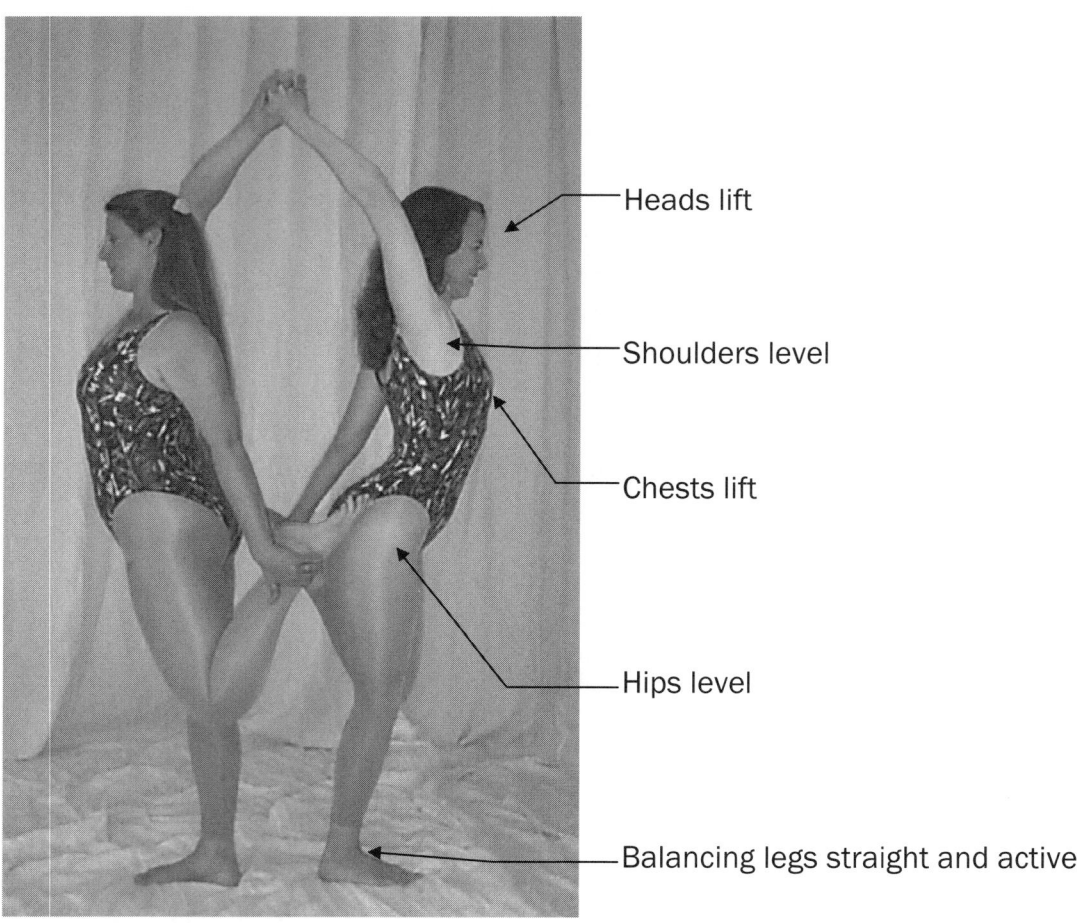

Heads lift

Shoulders level

Chests lift

Hips level

Balancing legs straight and active

Devotion - Feel the sense of lightness and upliftedness.

King's Dancer 2 (Natarajasana 2)

Intermediate/Advanced Levels

Cautions - If you feel you are going to fall, do NOT grab your partner or hold on to them to keep from falling!
- If you feel your Partner is going to fall, LET them fall and catch themselves without interference.

Instructions

1. Start standing front to front two to three feet apart (the exact distance will be determined by the balancing abilities of the least experienced Partner).
2. Bend the LEFT leg at the knee and grasp the front of the ankle with the LEFT hand.
3. Reach up and touch RIGHT hands palm to palm.

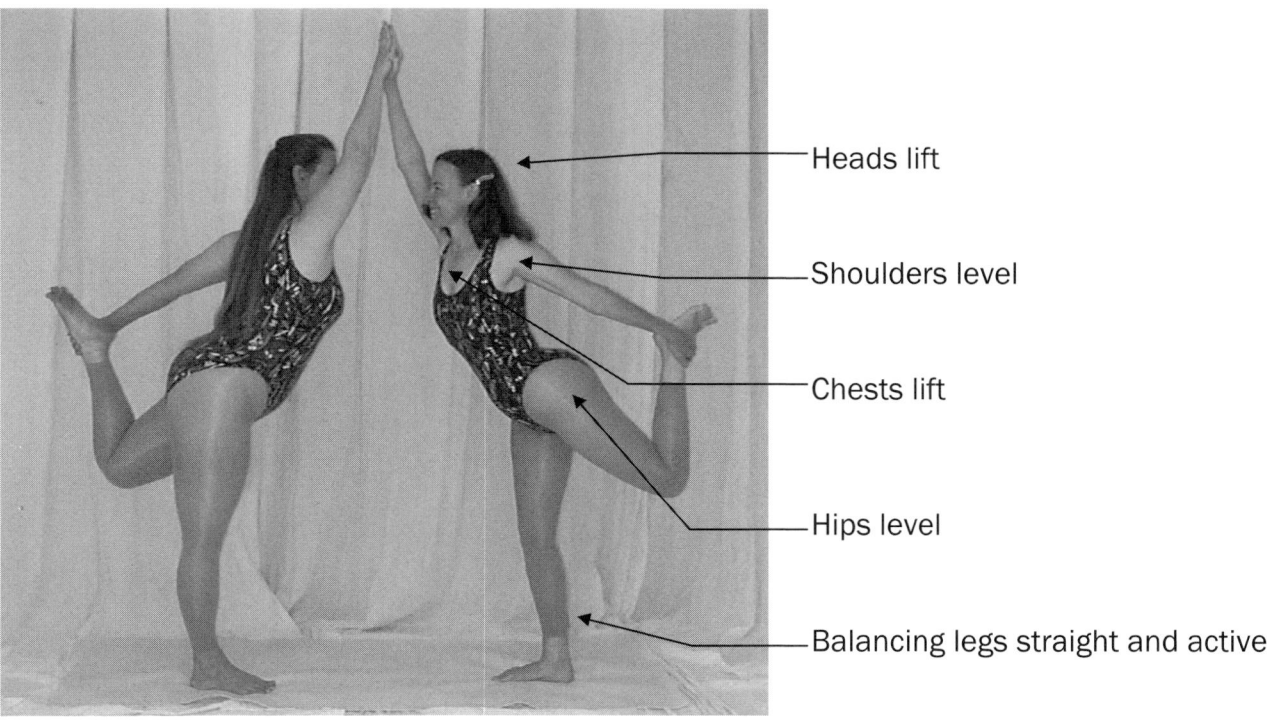

Heads lift

Shoulders level

Chests lift

Hips level

Balancing legs straight and active

Learning Another's Dance

Upward Facing Dog, Standing (Sama Adhomukha Svanasana)

All Levels

Instructions
1. Start standing face-to-face, with the tips of the big toes touching.
2. Clasp wrists.
3. Lift chests and lean back into the Standing Upward Facing Dog Pose.

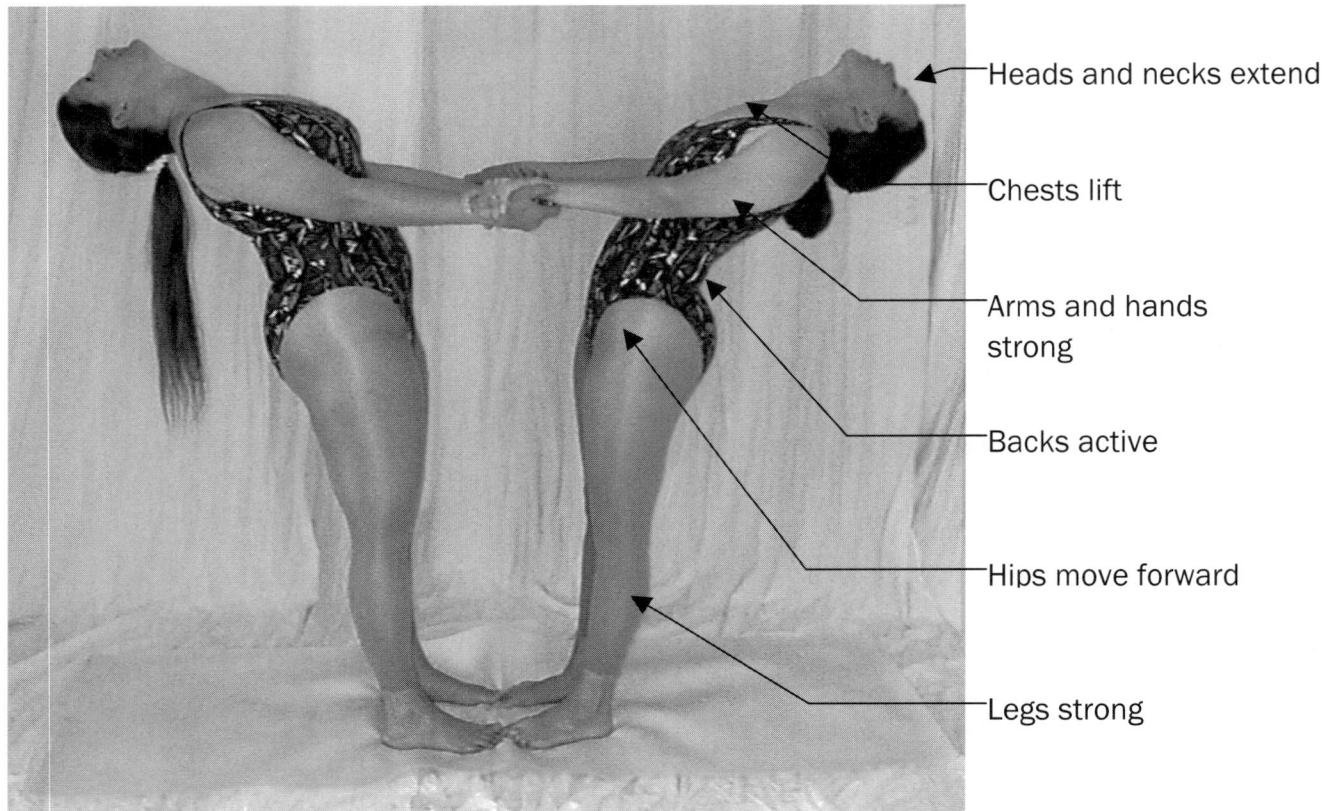

Chakra Explosion !

Chair (Utkatasana)

All Levels

Cautions - If you feel you are going to fall, do NOT grab your partner or hold on to them to keep from falling!

     - If you feel your Partner is going to fall, LET them fall and catch themselves without interference.

Instructions

1. Start sitting back to back on the floor .
2. Bend legs at the knees and place feet hip width with heel approximately one hand length from hips.
3. Push into one another's backs and rise to a "sitting" position.
4. Stretch arms over head and clasp hands.

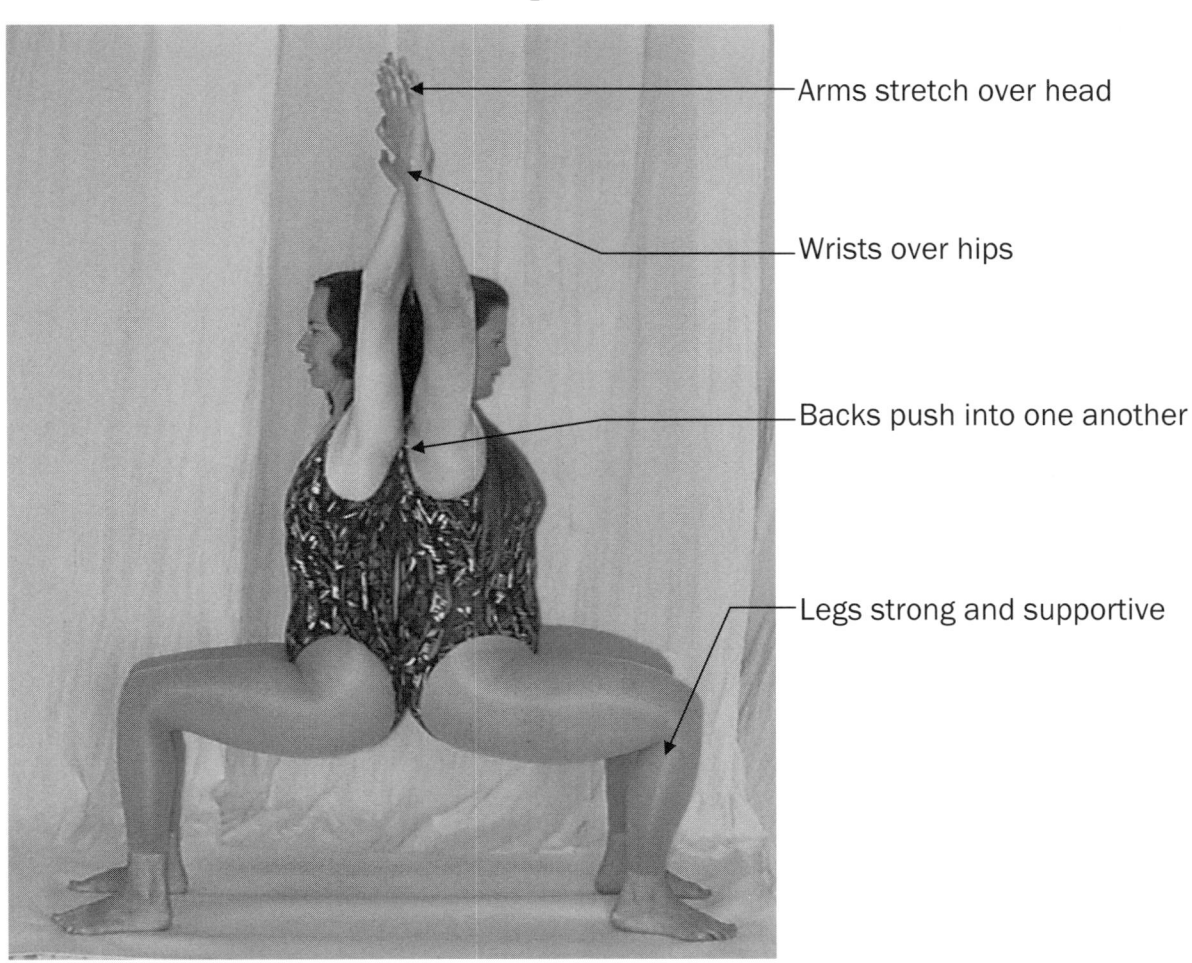

— Arms stretch over head

— Wrists over hips

— Backs push into one another

— Legs strong and supportive

Surprise! Easy Chair - Ahhh

Cross Gate (Parighasana 1)

All Levels

Cautions - If you feel you are going to fall, do NOT grab your partner or hold on to them to keep from falling!
- If you feel your Partner is going to fall, LET them fall and catch themselves without interference.

Instructions
1. Start facing front kneeling on the floor 4 - 6' apart (the exact distance will be determined by both Partner's leg length).
2. Extend INSIDE legs towards the center until soles of feet meet.
3. Stretch arms up over head and engage quadriceps in the legs.
4. Stretch torsos sideways from the hips towards the center and clasp hands.

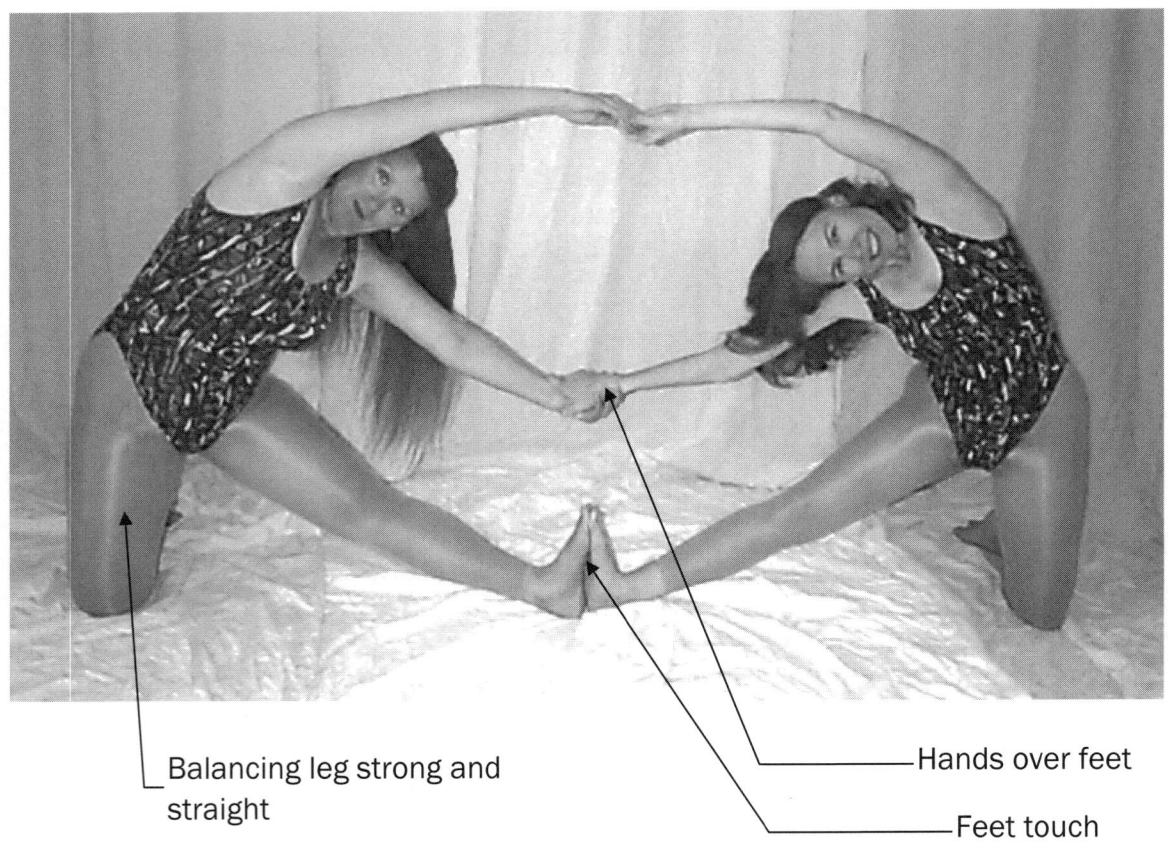

Balancing leg strong and straight

Hands over feet

Feet touch

Open Gate

Gate Latch Pose (Parighanasa 2)

All Levels

Cautions - If you feel you are going to fall, do NOT grab your partner or hold on to them to keep from falling!
- If you feel your Partner is going to fall, LET them fall and catch themselves without interference.

Instructions
1. Start facing front kneeling on the floor hips touching.
2. Extend OUTSIDE legs towards the outside.
3. Stretch arms up over head and engage quadriceps in the legs.
4. Stretch sideways from the hips towards the outside, stretch torsos towards the outside, clasp inside arms and reach outside hands towards feet.

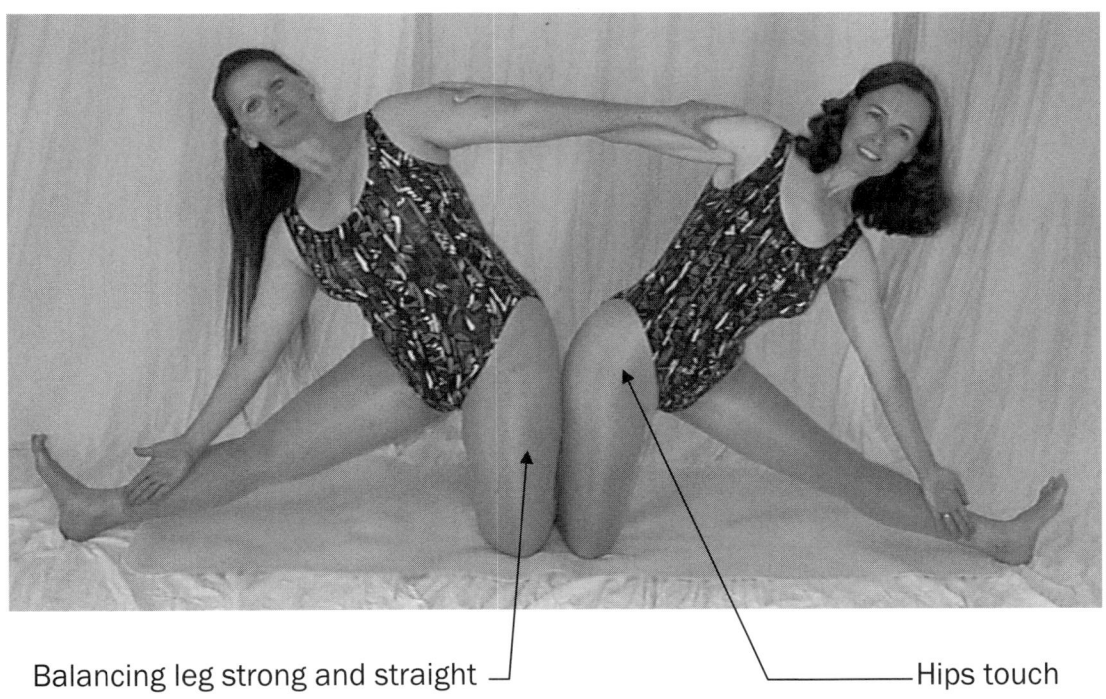

Balancing leg strong and straight ⌐   ⌐ Hips touch

Close Gate

Other Standing Poses

The following is a list of poses where at least one Partner stands during the pose or during one part of the pose:

Arm-Supported Backbend & Forward Pull Vinyasa (Figurehead Pose,
      Uttanasna, & Virbhadrasana II) - page 84
Back Stretcher (Utkatasana & Sitting Backbend) - page 86
Blue Moon (Uttanasana 1) - page 60
Blue Moon, Moving (Uttanasana 1, Moving) - page 61
Cheek to Cheek (Uttanasana 2) - page 62
Cheek to Cheek, Moving (Uttanasana 2, Moving) - page 63
Flying Cobra (Bujangasana 4) - page 90
Hang the Yogi (Uttanasana & Gajasana to Tadasana) - page 94
Hang the Yoga for 3 or More (Uttanasana & Adhomukha Svasana to Tadasana) -
      page 121
Torso Lift (Savasana & Tadasana) - page 108
Touching Hearts - page 124

HEADSTANDS

&

SHOULDERSTANDS

Back to Back Headstand 1 (Sirsasana 1)

Intermediate/Advanced Levels

Cautions - If you feel you are going to fall, calmly tell your Partner, tuck your knees into your chest, come out of the headstand, and move away them.

- If you feel your Partner is going to fall or they tell you they are going to fall, tell them you are going to come out and do as instructed above.

- You should be thoroughly familiar with the headstand before attempting this pose.

Instructions
1. Start in Child's Pose* facing head to head with 6-8" between the Partners' heads.
2. Both Partners move together into the Headstand one stage, at a time.

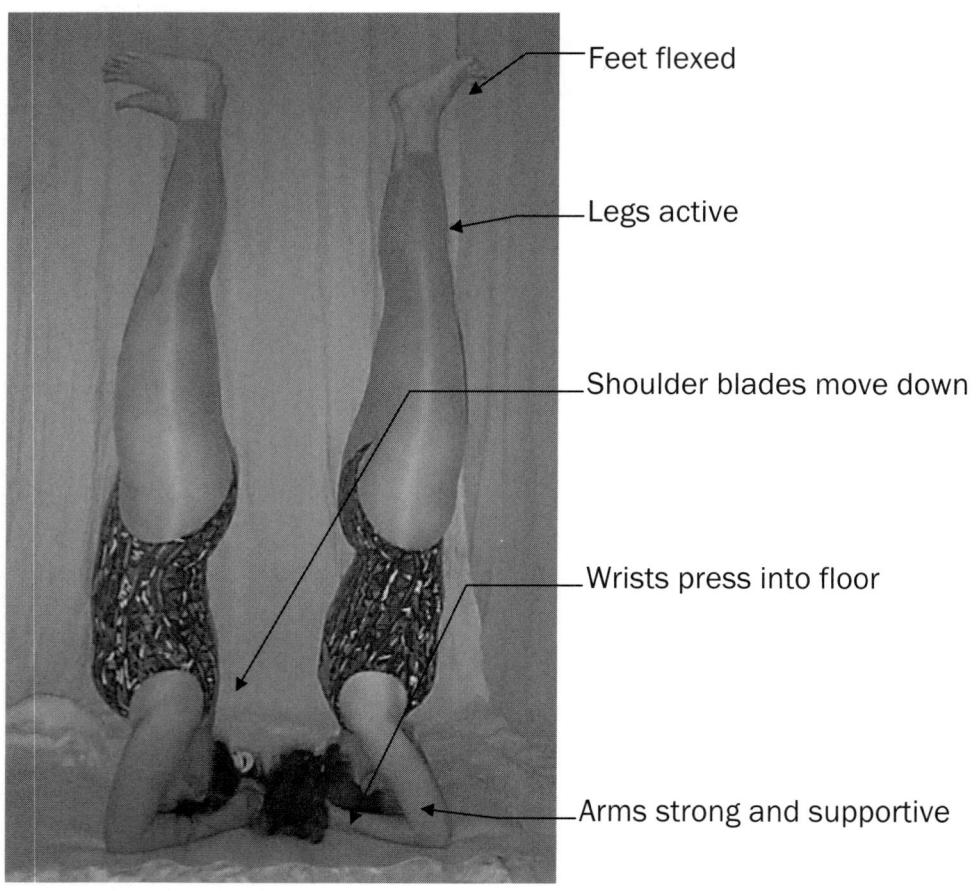

Feet flexed

Legs active

Shoulder blades move down

Wrists press into floor

Arms strong and supportive

Watching Each Other's Backs

* - See page 102 for a picture of Child's Pose

40

Front to Front Headstand (Sirsasana 2)

Advanced Level

Cautions - If you feel you are going to fall, calmly tell your Partner, spread your legs wide, and roll away from them.

- If you feel your Partner is going to fall or they tell you they are going to fall, tell them you will come out too and do as instructed above.
- You should be thoroughly familiar with the headstand and the split-leg headstand before attempting this pose.

Instructions

1. Start with Partner 1 in a Headstand.
2. Partner 2 stands in front of Partner 1's front side facing away from them, legs in a 4 1/2' wide or wider stance.
3. Partner 2 bends forward from the hips, being very careful not to bump Partner 1, places crown of head on the floor, and moves arms into headstand position.
4. Partner 2 moves into a headstand with legs spread apart by raising legs, then brings legs together over head. To come out, reverse the movements you used to get into the poses.

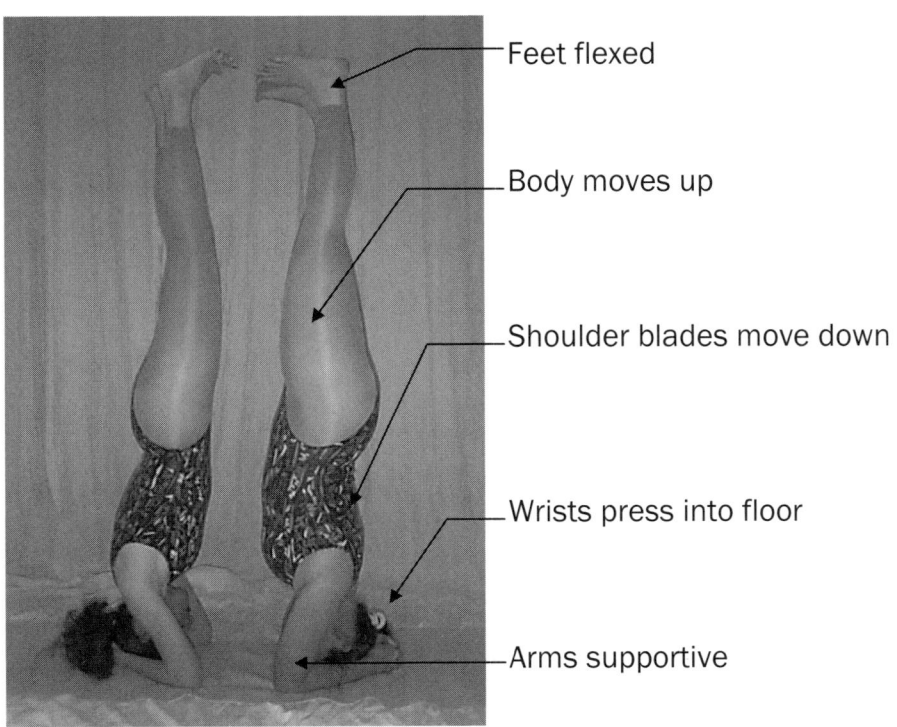

Feet flexed

Body moves up

Shoulder blades move down

Wrists press into floor

Arms supportive

Staring Mortality in the Face.

41

Back to Back Headstand Arch (Sirsasana 3)

Intermediate/Advanced Levels

Cautions - If you feel you are going to fall, calmly tell your Partner, tuck your knees into your chest, come out of the headstand, and move away from them.
- If you feel your Partner is going to fall or they tell you they are going to fall, tell them you will come out too and do as instructed above.
- You should be thoroughly familiar with the headstand before attempting this pose.

Instructions
1. Start in Child's Pose* facing head to head with 1 - 2' between the Partners' heads.
2. Both Partners move together into the Headstand one stage at a time.
3. Partner 1 Bends RIGHT leg at the knee and places the sole of their foot on their LEFT knee. Partner 2 mirrors with their LEFT foot.
4. Partners touch RIGHT and LEFT feet as shown.

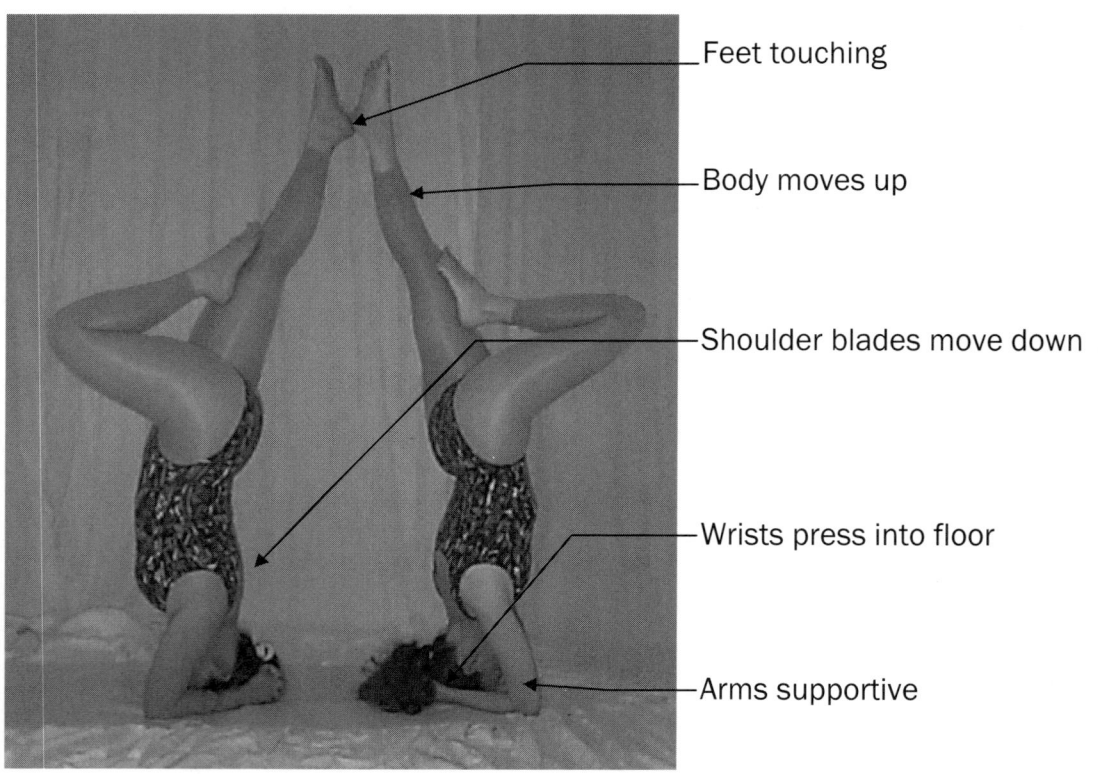

Feet touching

Body moves up

Shoulder blades move down

Wrists press into floor

Arms supportive

Sole to Soul

* - See Page 102 for picture of the Child's Pose

Shoulderstand and Squatting Pose 1 (Sarvangasana & Squat 1)

All Levels

Cautions - Do not pull your partner any farther than is comfortable for them.
- You should be thoroughly familiar with the shoulderstand before attempting this pose.

Instructions

1. Start with Partner 1 in a full Shoulderstand and Partner 2 in a Sitting Squat with Partners facing back to back.
2. Partner 2 moves backward to Partner 1 and supports Partner 1 with their back.
3. Partner 2 takes Partner 1's arms by the wrist and VERY gently pulls on Partner 1's arms. Partners coordinate breath.
4. To adjust the pose or provide more support for Partner 1, Partner 2 rounds their back down, then sits up straight while keeping in contact with Partner 1's back.

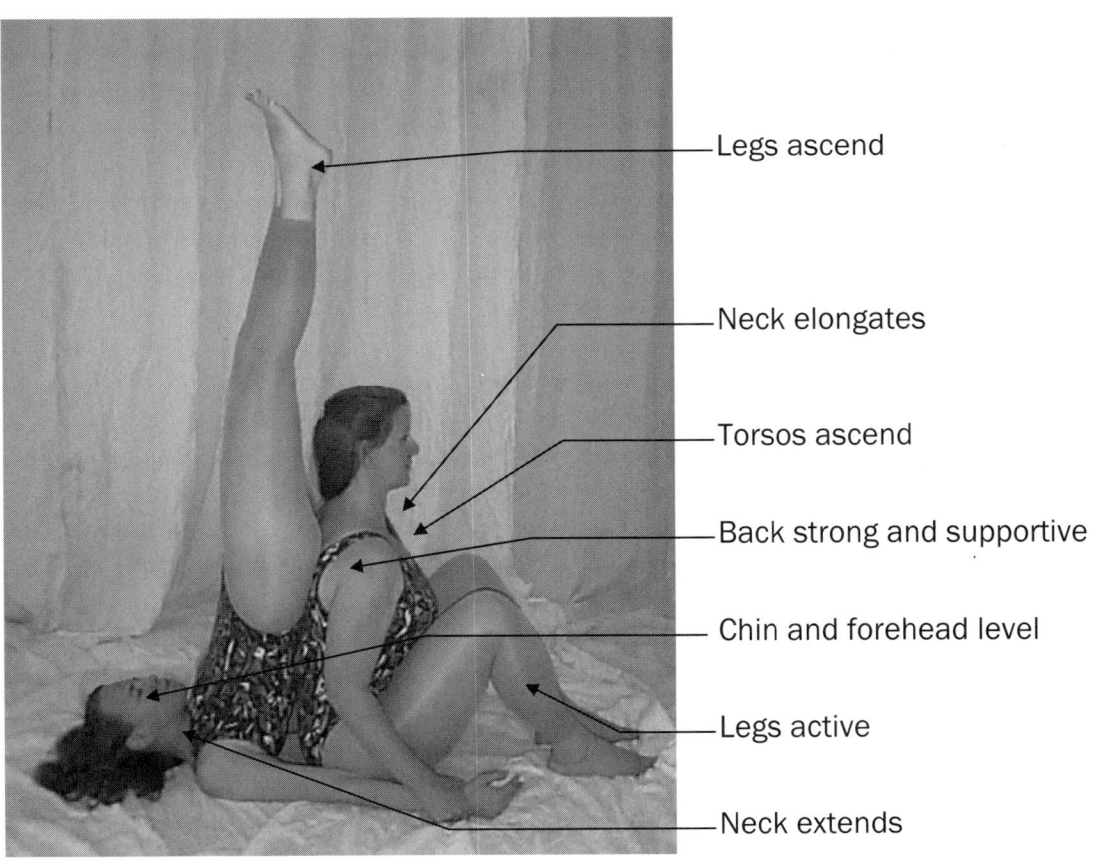

Legs ascend

Neck elongates

Torsos ascend

Back strong and supportive

Chin and forehead level

Legs active

Neck extends

Learning how to support and be supported.

Shoulderstand and Squatting Pose 2 (Sarvangasana & Squat 2)

Advanced Level

Cautions - Do not pull your partner any farther than is comfortable for them.
- You should be thoroughly familiar with the shoulderstand before attempting this pose.

Instructions
1. Start with Partner 1 in a full Shoulderstand and Partner 2 in a Sitting Squat with Partners facing back to back.
2. Partner 2 moves backward to Partner 1 and supports Partner 1 with their back.
3. Partner 2 takes Partner 1's arms and wraps them around Partner 2's shins. Partners coordinate breath.
4. To adjust the pose to provide more support for Partner 1, Partner 2 rounds their back down, then sits up straight while keeping in contact with Partner 1's back.

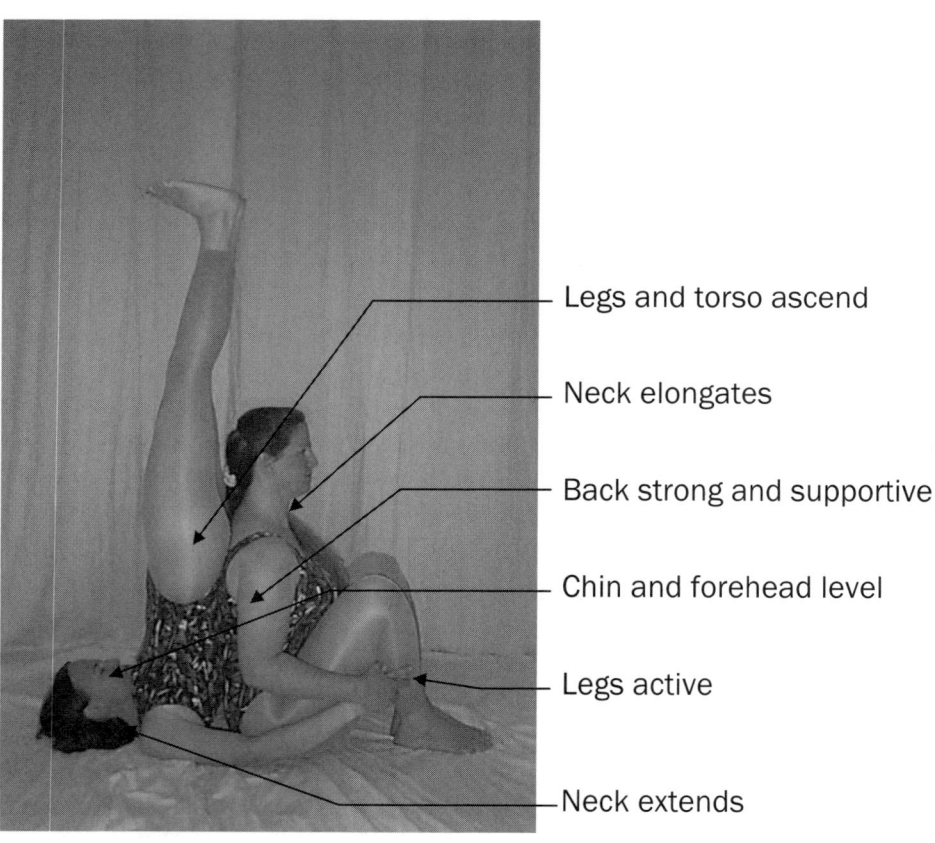

Legs and torso ascend

Neck elongates

Back strong and supportive

Chin and forehead level

Legs active

Neck extends

Farthering the support.

Steeple Tower (Ardha Sarvangasana)

All Levels

Instructions
1. Start lying crown to crown, face up, flat on the floor.
2. Each Partner moves into a Half Shoulderstand.
3. Touch toes.

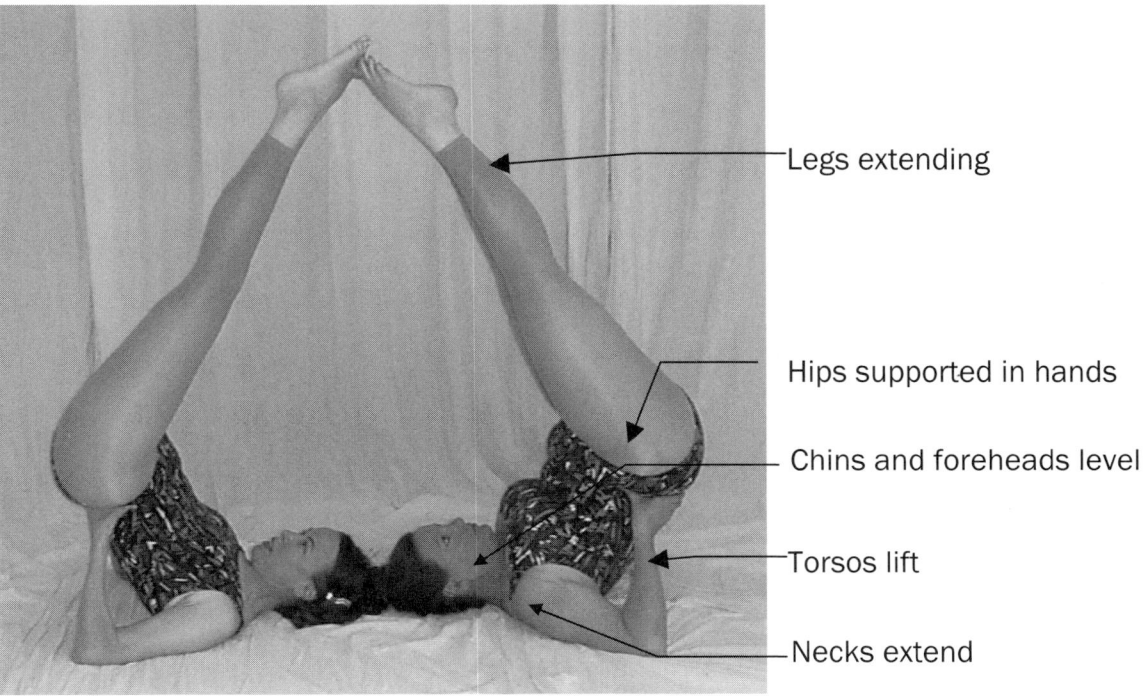

Legs extending

Hips supported in hands

Chins and foreheads level

Torsos lift

Necks extend

Lofty High

Steeple Spire (Salamba Sarvangasana)

Intermediate/Advanced Levels

Instructions

1. Start with Partners lying toe to toe on their backs with their legs bent at the knees and their feet flat on the floor.
2. Move into shoulderstands.
3. Partners match feet on each side.

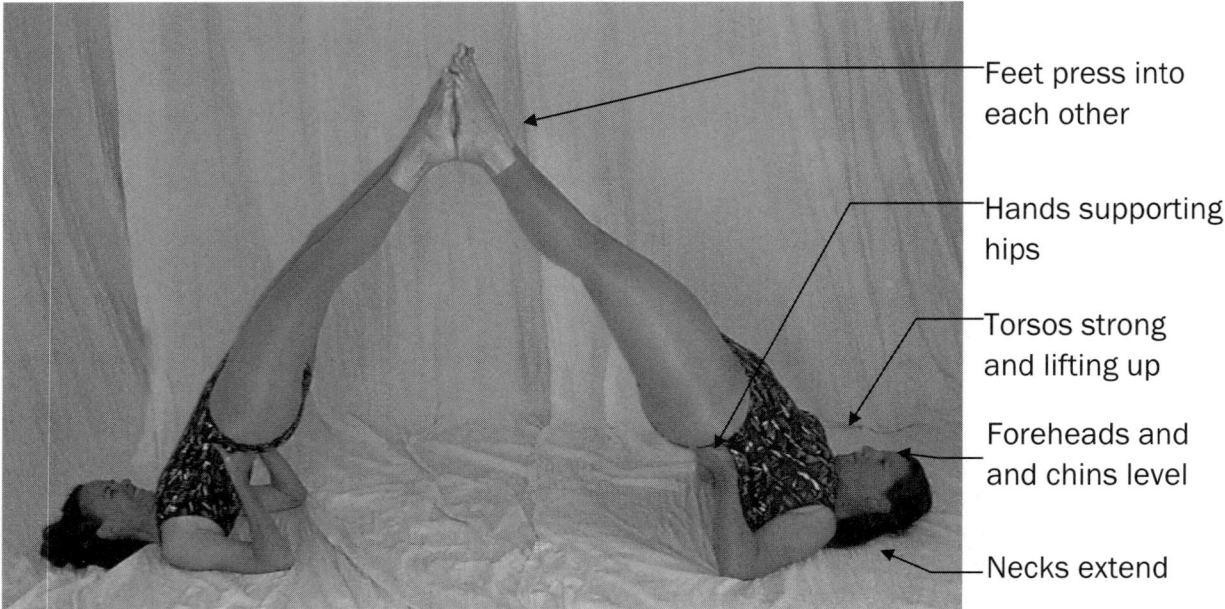

Ending at a Point

Steeple Bell (Eka PadaViparita Karani)

Intermediate/Advanced Levels

Instructions

1. Start with Partners lying toe to toe on their backs with their legs bent at the knees and their feet flat on the floor.
2. Move into shoulderstands.
3. Partners match feet on one side.
4. Place other foot on kneecap of the oposite leg as shown.

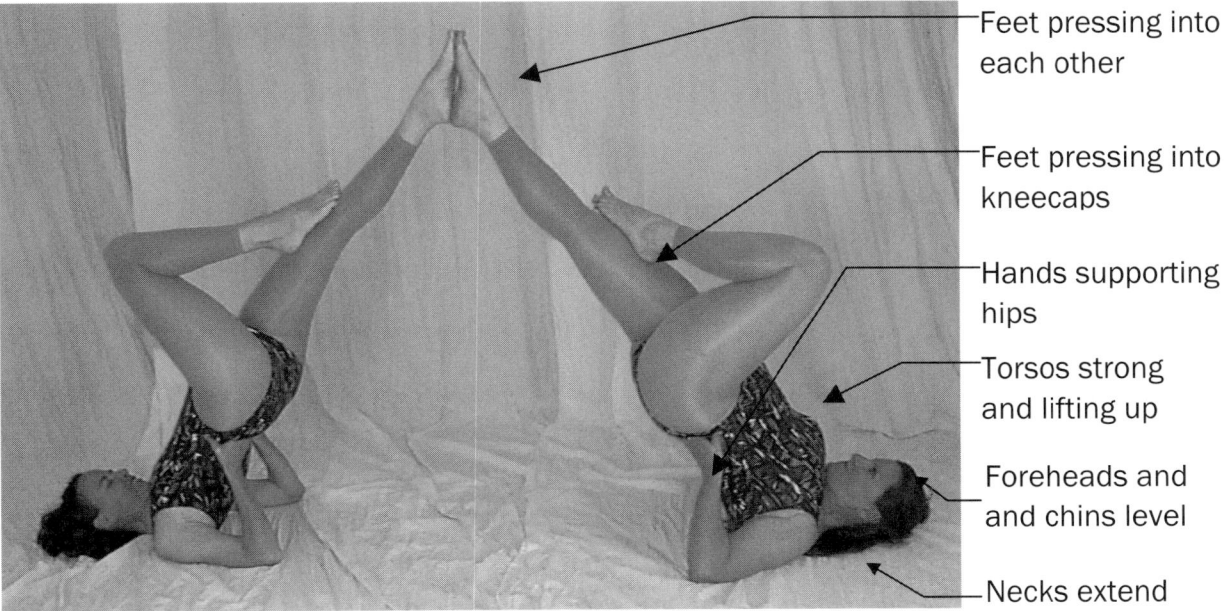

Containing the Chime

Other Inverted Poses

The following is a list of poses where at least one Partner is inverted or up side down during the pose or during one part of the pose:

FISH POSES

Side by Side Fish (Ardha Matsyasana 1)

All Levels

Instructions
1. Start with Partners lying on their backs side by side, hip to hip, and legs pointing in opposite directions.
2. Each Partner moves into the Fish Pose.

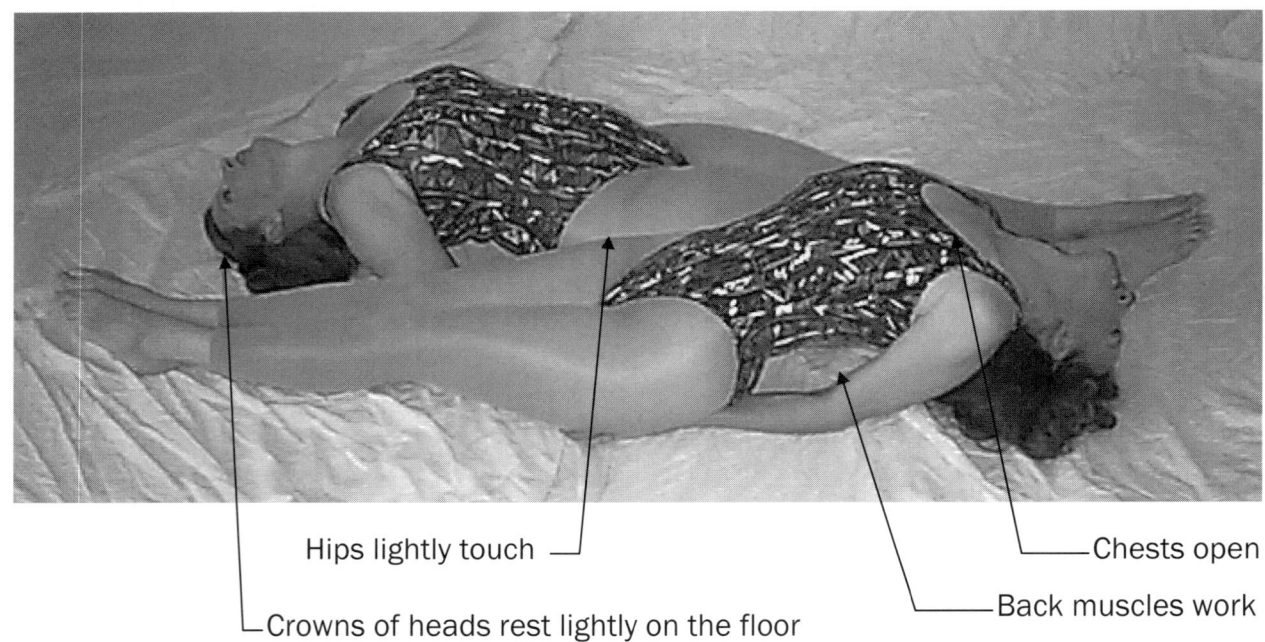

Hips lightly touch ⏌

⎿Crowns of heads rest lightly on the floor

⎾Chests open

⎿Back muscles work

Hearts Afloat

Knee to Knee Fish (Ardha Matsyasana 2)

All Levels

Instructions

1. Start with Partners lying on their backs knee to knee with legs in the Cross Legged Pose as shown (Beginning) or
2. in the Easy Pose* (Intermediate) or
3. in the Lotus Pose* (Advanced).
4. Each Partner places their hands under their hips, pushes against the other's knees, and moves into the Fish Pose.

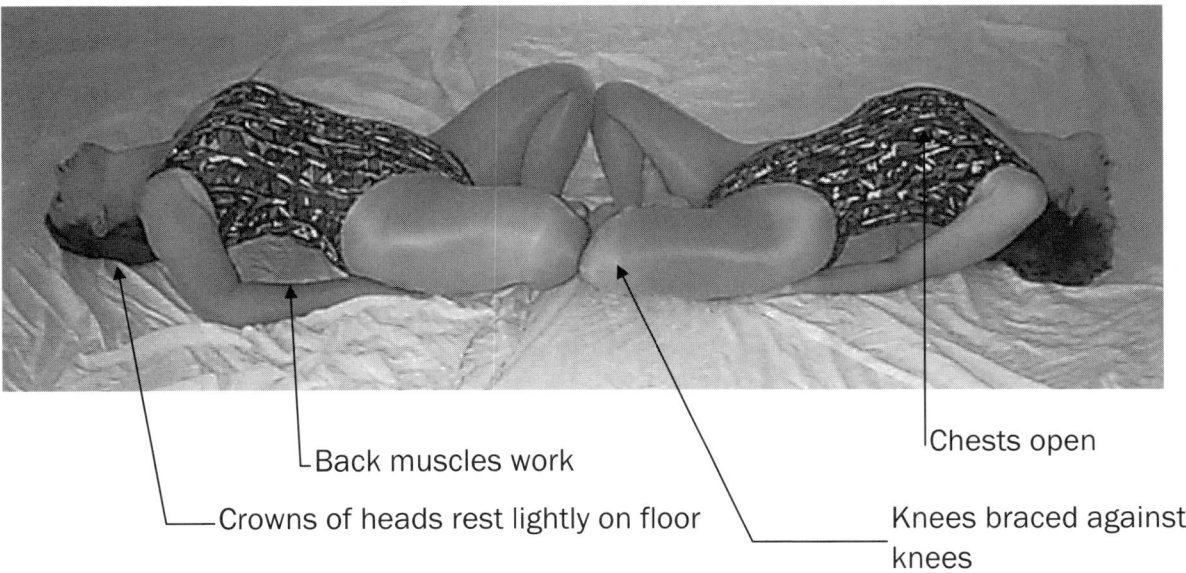

Back muscles work

Crowns of heads rest lightly on floor

Chests open

Knees braced against knees

Two Boats Moored Together

* See Index or Table of Contents for more information on the Easy Pose and the Lotus Pose

Yogi on Board (Ardha Matsyasana & Balasana 1)

All Levels

Instructions
1. Start with Partner 1 in Child's Pose.
2. Partner 2 sits LIGHTLY on Partner 1's coccyx facing away from Partner 1.
3. Partner 2 stretches out legs and rests feet or heel on the floor behind Partner 1.
4. Partner 2 moves into a backbend resting on Partner 1's back. Partners grasp hands and breathe together.

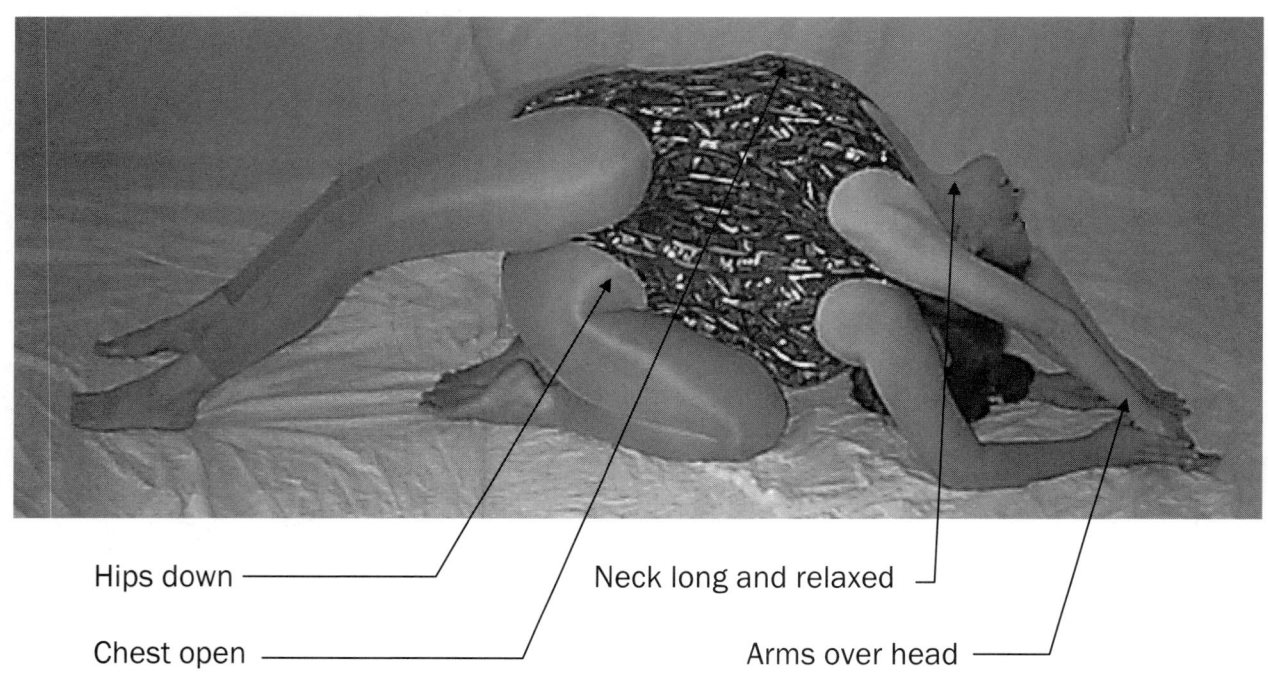

Hips down ——————

Chest open ——————

Neck long and relaxed ⏐

Arms over head ——————

Child Under Bridge

Sitting Forward Bend/Backbend 1
(Paschimottanasana & Ardha Matsyasana 1)

All Levels

Instructions
1. Start with Partners sitting back to back with legs stretched out in front of them.
2. Partner 2 moves into a backbend resting on Partner 1's back.
3. Partner 1 gently pulls Partner 2's arms straight out from shoulders. Breathe together.

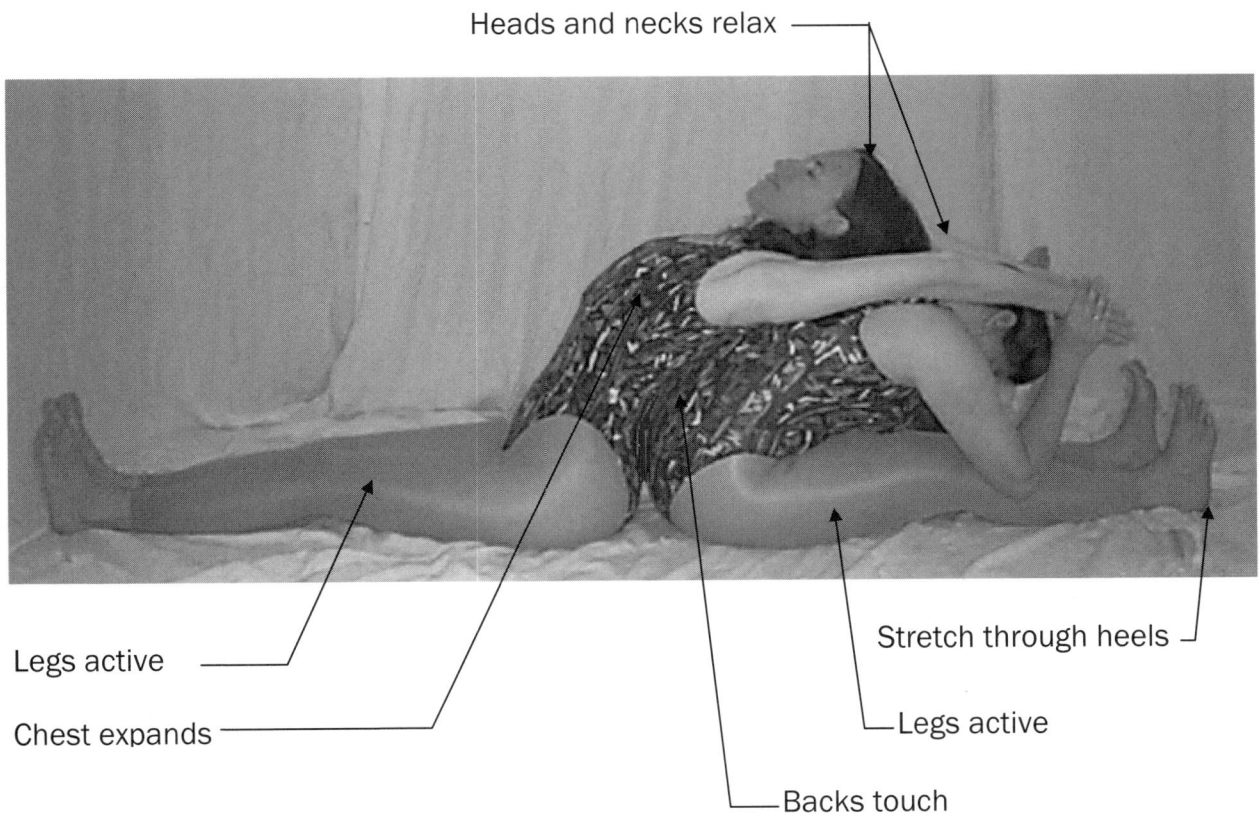

Heads and necks relax

Legs active

Chest expands

Stretch through heels

Legs active

Backs touch

Open and Surrender

Sitting Forward Bend/Backbend 2
(Paschimottanasana & Ardha Matsyasana 2)

Intermediate/Advanced Levels

Instructions
1. Start with Partner 1 in a Sitting Forward Bend.
2. Partner 2 sits lightly on Partner 1's lower back.
3. Partner 2 carefully moves into a backbend resting on Partner 1's back and their head resting on Partner 1's head.
4. Partners clasp hands and Partner 1 pulls gently on Partner 2's arms..

Heads and necks relaxed

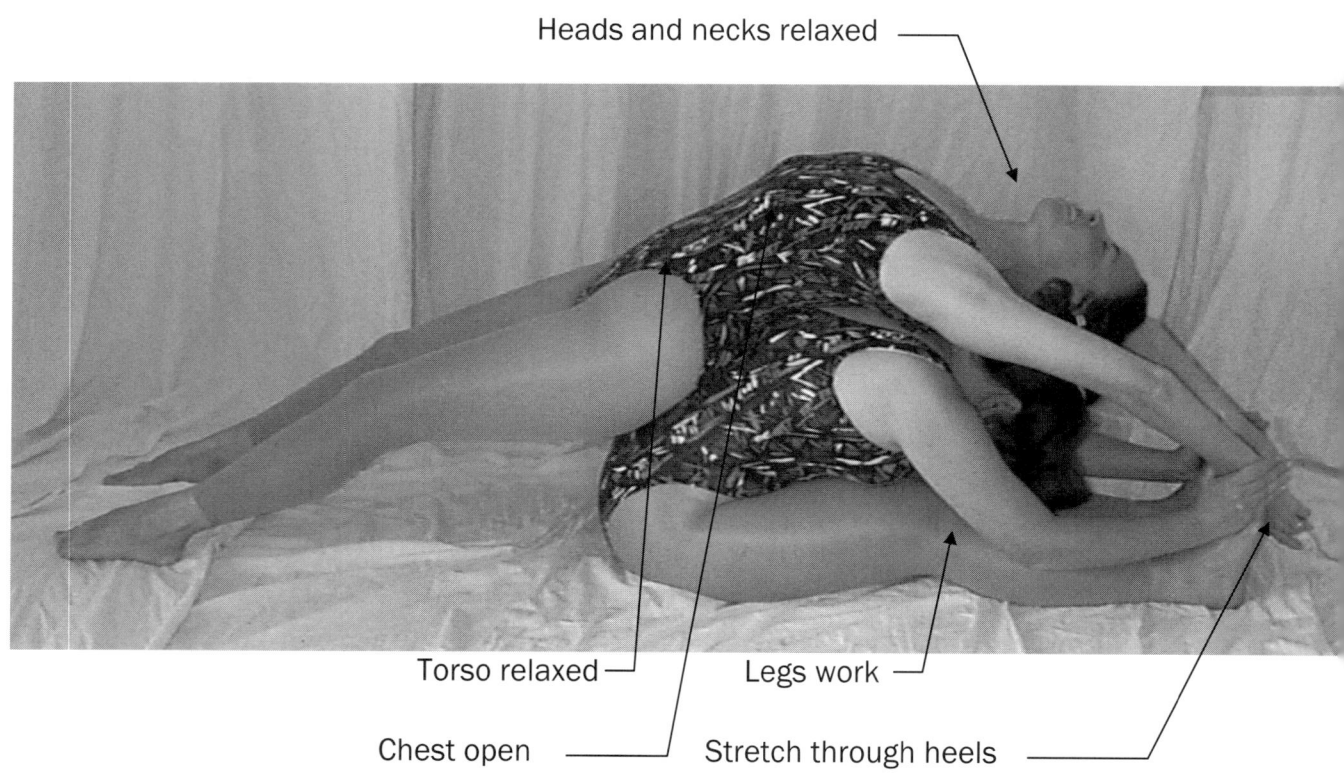

Torso relaxed

Chest open

Legs work

Stretch through heels

Protection and Exposure

Fish & Child's Pose (Ardha Matsyasana & Balasana 2)

Advanced Level

Cautions - The Partner in the Child's Pose **MUST** be flexible enough for their hips to rest on their heels, torso to rest on their thighs, and head to rest on the floor. This will help them avoid injury to their hips, back, and knees. Also, their back **MUST** be evenly rounded (side to side and front to back) to properly support the Partner doing the Fish Pose.

Instructions
1. Start with Partner 1 in Child's Pose (correct pose).
2. Partner 2 squats with their lower back against Partner 1's waist.
3. Partner 2 Positions one hand on the upper thoracic part of Partner 1's spine and their other hand on the lower lumbar and moves into the Fish Pose across the top of Partner 1's back.

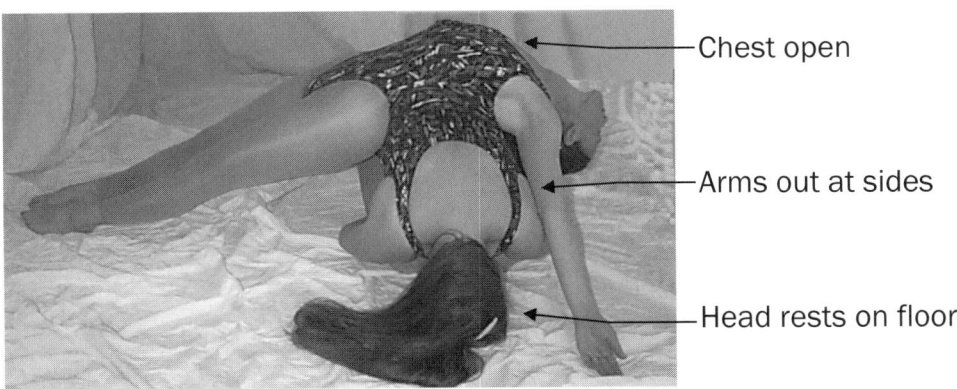

Chest open

Arms out at sides

Head rests on floor

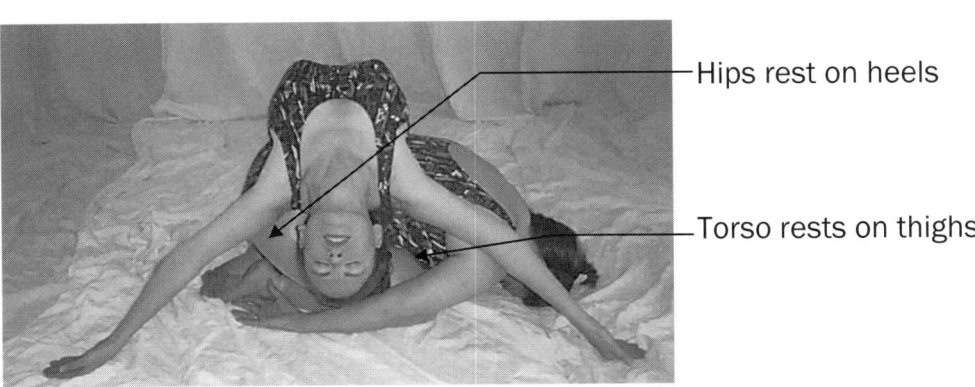

Hips rest on heels

Torso rests on thighs

Expansion and Support

55

FORWARD BENDS

The Suspension Bridge (Parsva Uttanasana 1)

All Levels

Caution - Keep arms muscles engaged during all phases of the pose.

Instructions
1. Start standing face to face and toes to toes.
2. Bend arms and the elbows, clasp wrists, and engage all the muscles in the arms.
3. Pull on each other's arms and slowly bend at the hips until arms are extended all the way.
4. To come out keep the tension in the arms, bend at the elbows and straighten bodies.

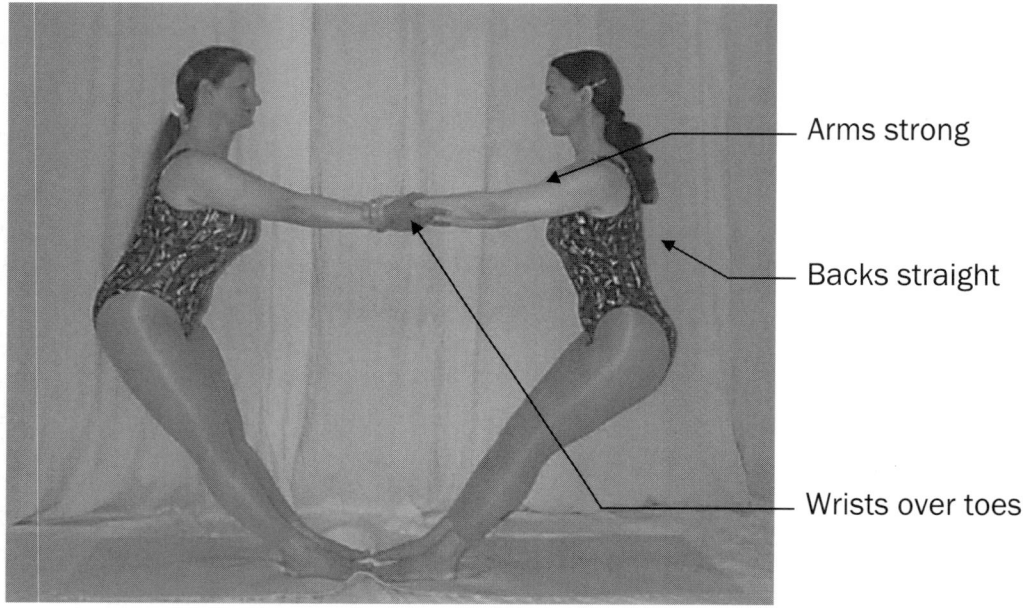

Putting Your "Back Side" into It

The Rope Extension Stretch (Parsva Uttanasana 2)

All Levels

Caution - Keep arm muscles engaged during all phases of the pose.

Instructions
1. Start by making a strong loop with a 6-8' yoga belt.
2. Slip the belt around hips and stand back to back with the belt taut.
3. Stretch arms over head and gently "lean" into the belt until you find a balance point with your Partner. If your legs are not straight, adjust the distance between the Partners.
4. To come out keep the tension in the arms, bend at the elbows and straighten bodies.

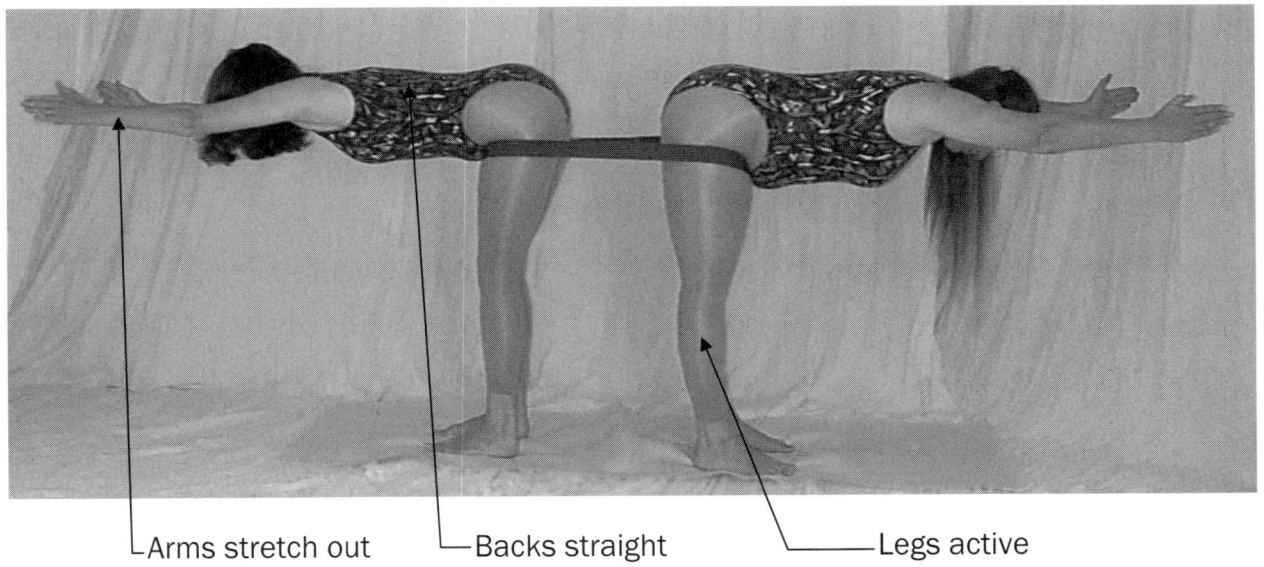

└Arms stretch out   └Backs straight   └Legs active

Suspended in Time

Blue Moon (Uttanasana 1)

All Levels

Caution - Do **NOT** pull yourself or your Partner any farther than is comfortable for your backs.

Instructions
1. Start standing back to back, feet 10-12" apart, gluteals touching.
2. INHALE while raising arms over heads, then EXHALE while bending forward from the hips with a straight torsos until torsos form a 90 degree angle with legs. Remain in this position for 3-4 breaths to let their hip muscles stretch and relax.
3. Then EXHALE, relax torsos down, . . .
4. . . . bring hands between legs, and grip one another's hands, forearms, or elbows. Coordinate breathing and **GENTLY** pull torsos towards one another with each EXHALE.

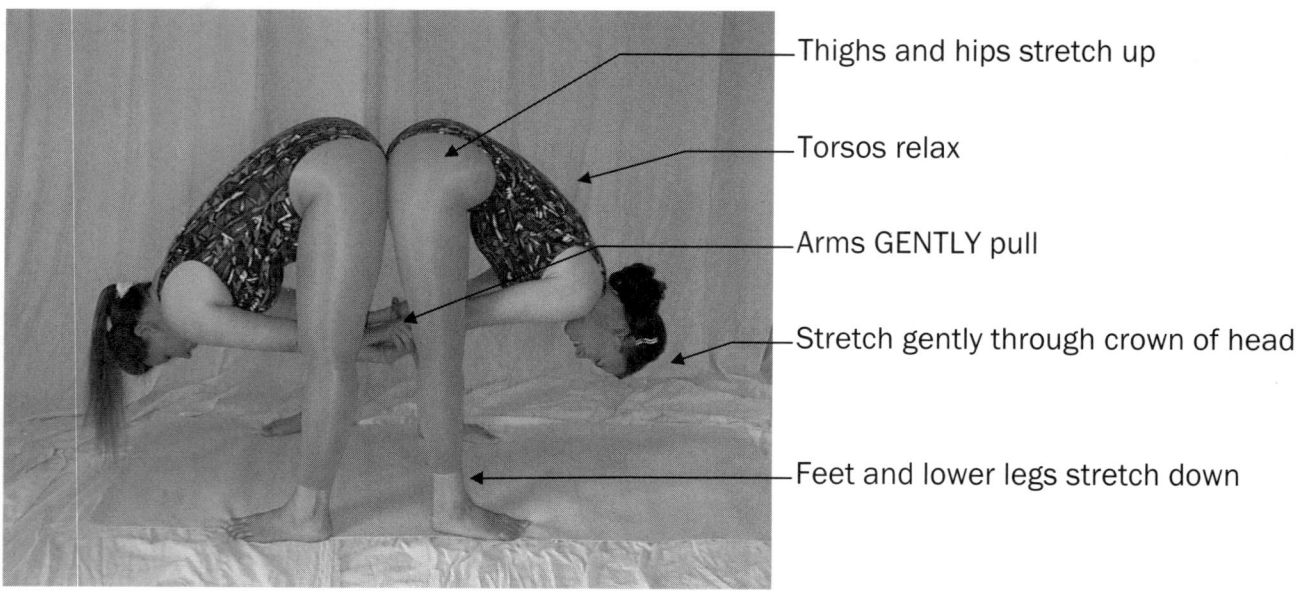

Thighs and hips stretch up

Torsos relax

Arms GENTLY pull

Stretch gently through crown of head

Feet and lower legs stretch down

Seeing Chipmunks

Blue Moon, Moving (Uttanasana 1, Moving)

All Levels

Caution - Do **NOT** pull yourself or your Partner any farther than is comfortable
for your backs.

Instructions
1. Start in the "Blue Moon" Pose.
2. Partners grasp hands and reverse coordinate their breathing.
3. Partner 1 EXHALES and leans forward as far as is comfortable while Partner 2
   INHALES and raises upper body up as far as it can comfortably go.
4. Then both Partners reverse the movement. Repeat gently and carefully for a
   total of 10 breaths.

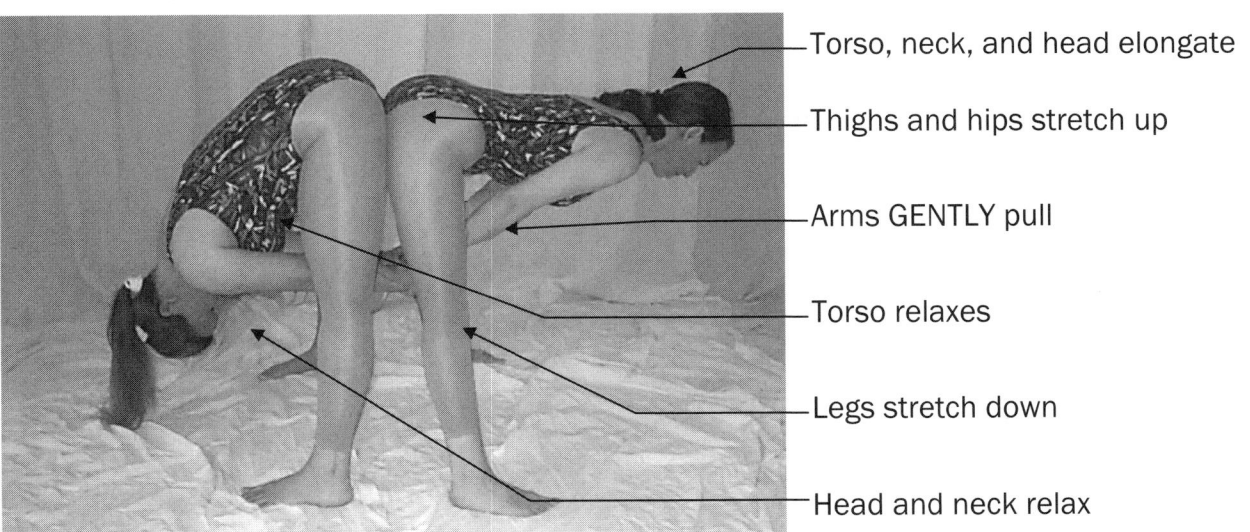

- Torso, neck, and head elongate
- Thighs and hips stretch up
- Arms GENTLY pull
- Torso relaxes
- Legs stretch down
- Head and neck relax

Breathing "In Counter"

Cheek to Cheek (Uttanasana 2)

All Levels

Caution - Do **NOT** pull yourself or your Partner any farther than is comfortable for your backs.

Instructions
1. Start standing back to back, feet 6-12" apart, gluteals touching.
2. INHALE while raising arms over heads, then EXHALE while bending forward from the hips with straight torsos until torsos form a 90 degree angle with legs. Remain in this position for 3-4 breaths to let hip muscles stretch and relax.
3. Then EXHALE, relax torsos down, . . .
4. . . . bring hands outside of legs, and grip one another's hands, forearms, or elbows. Coordinate breathing and **GENTLY** pull torsos towards one another with each EXHALE.

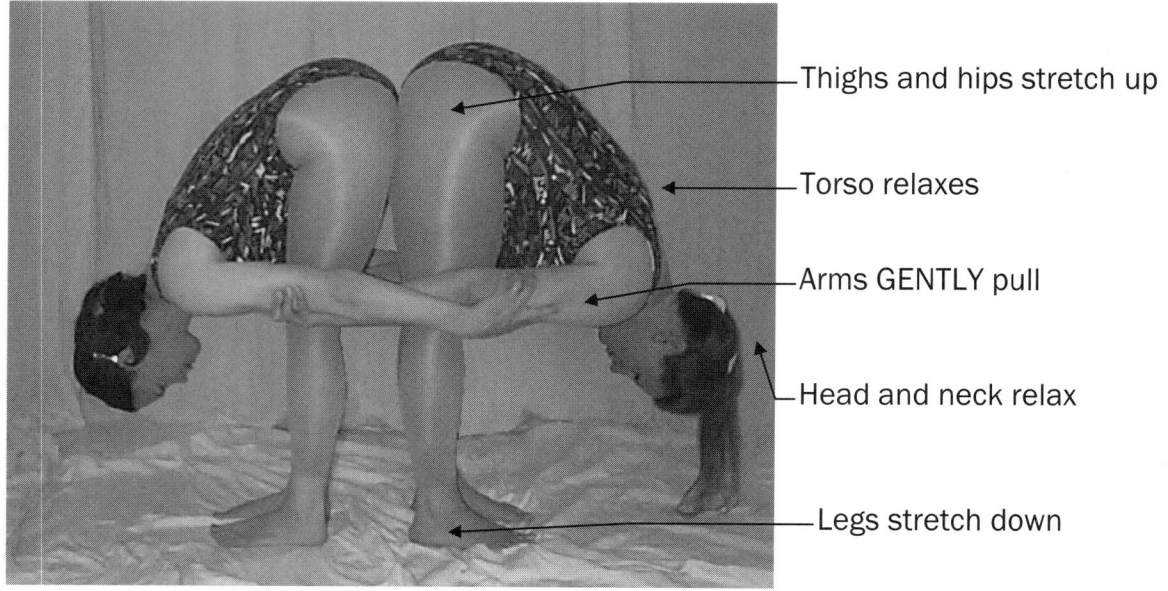

Thighs and hips stretch up

Torso relaxes

Arms GENTLY pull

Head and neck relax

Legs stretch down

Feeling the Heat

Cheek to Cheek, Moving (Uttanasana 2, Moving)

All Levels

Caution - Do **NOT** pull yourself or your Partner any farther than is comfortable for your backs.

Instructions
1. Start in the "Cheek to Cheek Pose".
2. Grasp Partner's hands and reverse coordinate breathing.
3. Partner 1 EXHALES and leans forward as far as is comfortable while Partner 2 INHALES and raises torso up as far as they comfortably can.
4. Then Partners reverse the movement. Repeat gently and carefully for a total of 10 breaths.

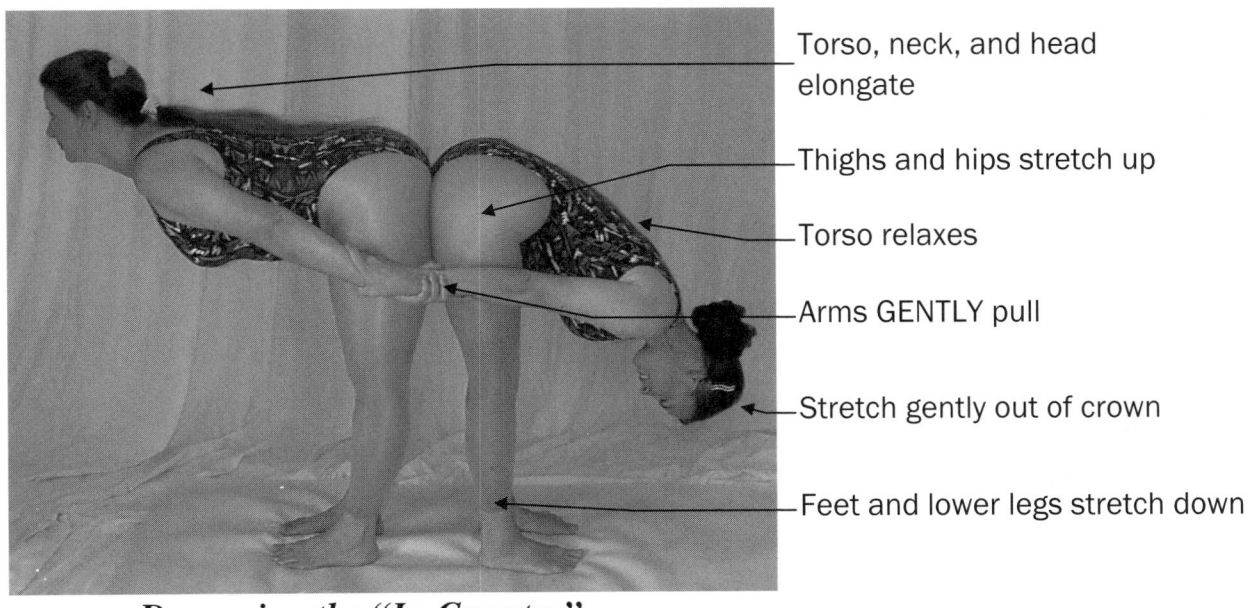

Torso, neck, and head elongate

Thighs and hips stretch up

Torso relaxes

Arms GENTLY pull

Stretch gently out of crown

Feet and lower legs stretch down

Deepening the "In Counter"

Ankle Lock (Uttanasana 3)

All Levels

Caution - Do **NOT** pull yourself or your Partner any farther than is comfortable for your backs.

Instructions
1. Start standing back to back, feet 6-12" apart, gluteals touching.
2. INHALE while raising arms over heads, then EXHALE while bending forward from the hips with straight torsos until torsos form a 90 degree angle with legs. Remain in this position for 3-4 breaths to let hip muscles stretch and relax.
3. Then EXHALE, relax torsos down.
4. Partners bring hands to grip one another's ankles and coordinate breathing.

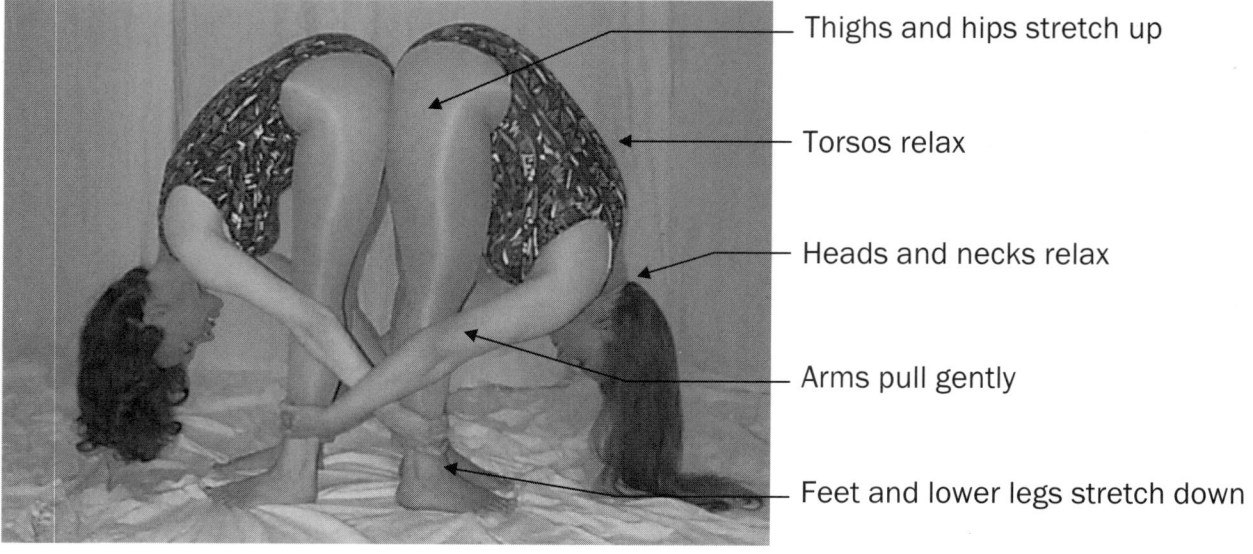

Thighs and hips stretch up

Torsos relax

Heads and necks relax

Arms pull gently

Feet and lower legs stretch down

Coming Closer Together

Foot Lock (Uttanasana 4)

All Levels

Caution - Do **NOT** pull yourself or your Partner any farther than is comfortable
for your backs.

Instructions
1. Start standing face to face, 1-2' apart.
2. Partner 1 INHALES while raising arms over head, then EXHALES while
   bending forward from the hips to a full forward bend.
3. Partner 2 does the same, being careful not to bump into Partner 1.
4. Partners bring hands to grip one another's feet and coordinate breathing.

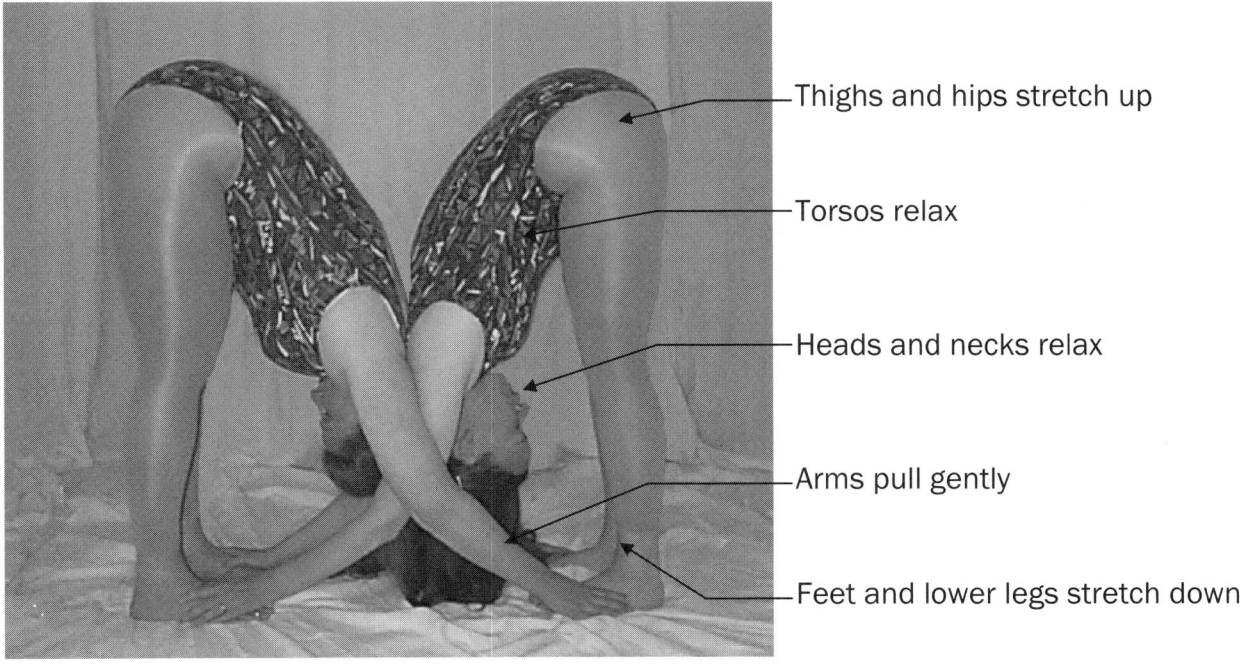

Thighs and hips stretch up

Torsos relax

Heads and necks relax

Arms pull gently

Feet and lower legs stretch down

Meeting of the Minds

Snowflake (Upavistha Konasana 2)

All Levels

Instructions
1. Start sitting back to back with gleutials, upperback, and shoulders touching.
2. Spread legs as far apart as is comfortable.
3. Reach back to lightly grasp the top of your Partners' thighs.
4. GENTLY pull Partners' legs to increase stretch.

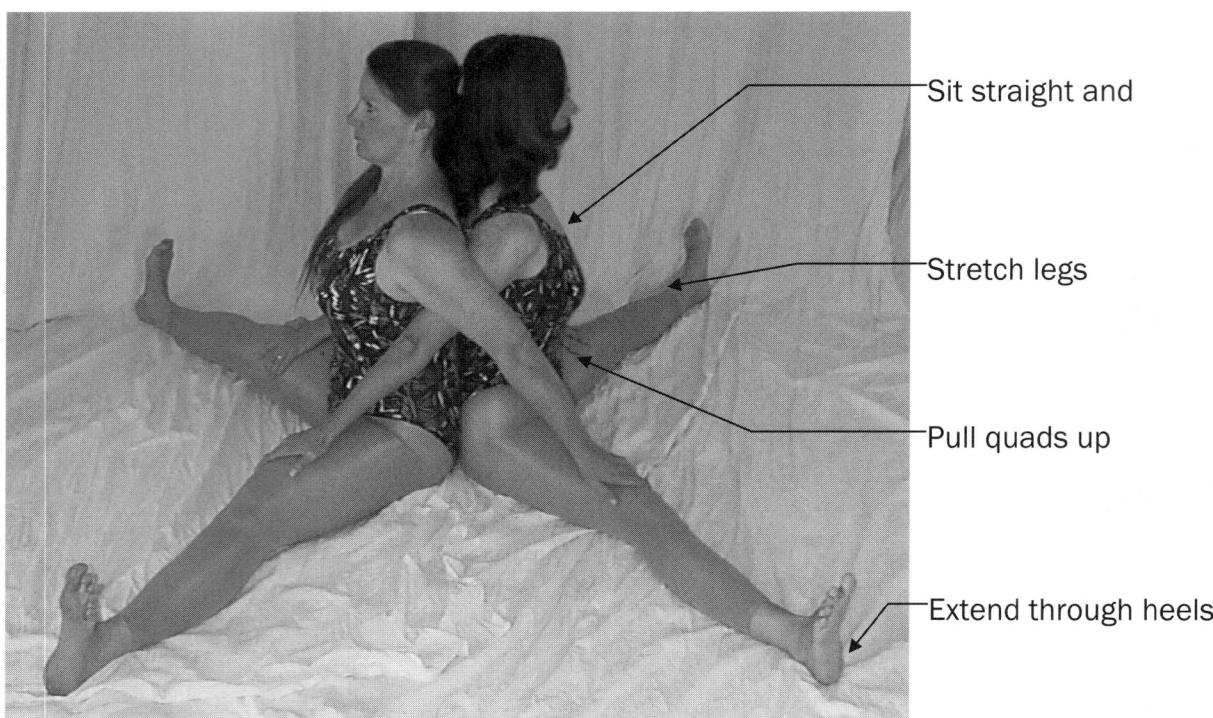

Sit straight and

Stretch legs

Pull quads up

Extend through heels

Alone Yet Supported

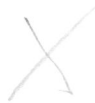

Legs Wide Stretch (Upavistha Konasana 3)

All Levels

Caution - Do **NOT** pull yourself or your Partner any farther than is comfortable for your legs.

Instructions
1. Start sitting face to face, feet to feet, legs spread as wide as is comfortable for the LESS flexible Partner.
2. Both Partners grasp each other's hands and begin to pull gently to stretch the legs a little wider.
3. Gaze into one another's eyes.

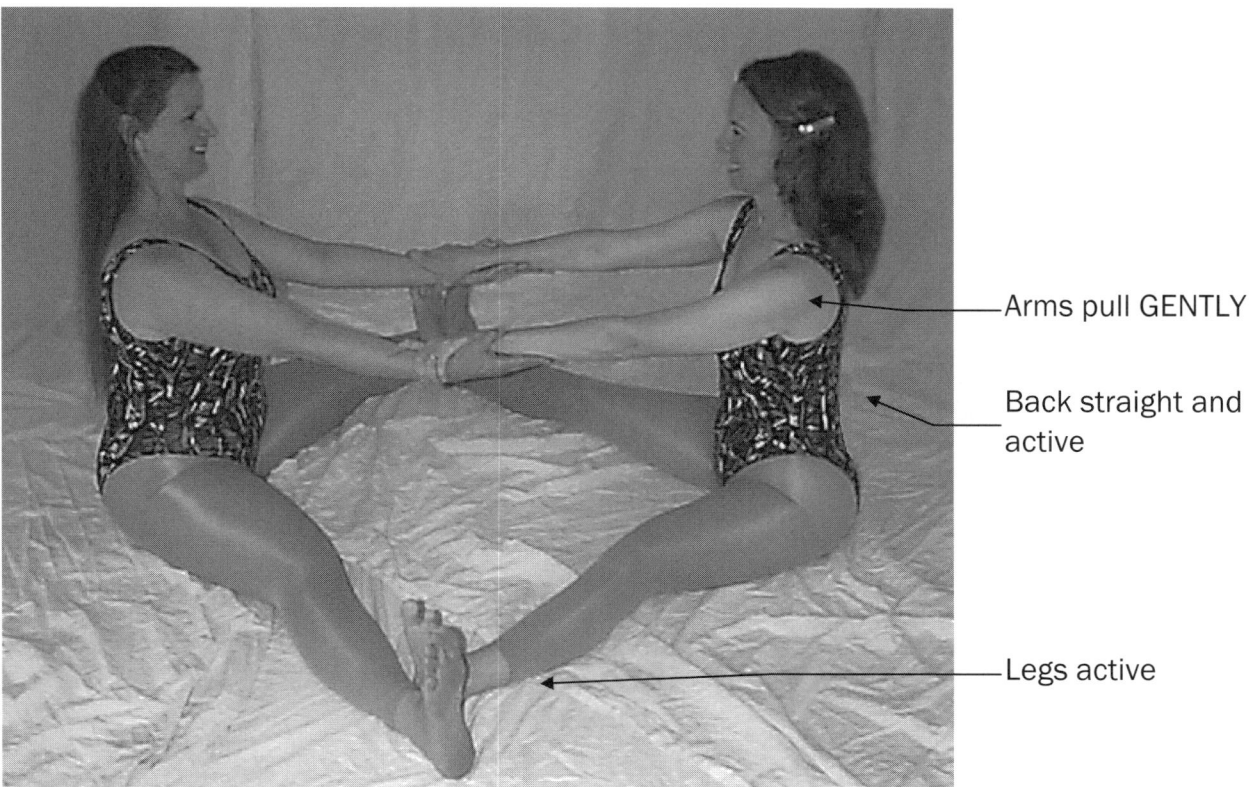

Arms pull GENTLY

Back straight and active

Legs active

Union

Sea-Saw 2 (Upavista Konasana 3, Moving)

All Levels

Caution - Do **NOT** pull yourself or your Partner any farther than is comfortable for your legs, back, and upper body.

Instructions

1. Start sitting face to face, feet to feet, with both Partners legs spread as wide as is comfortable for each. The LESS flexible Partner places the soles of their feet on the inside of the MORE flexible Partner's legs.
2. Both Partners grasp each other's hands and reverse coordinate their breathing.
3. Partner 1 EXHALES and leans forward as far as they comfortably can while Partner 2 INHALES and sits up as far as they can.
4. Then both Partner reverse the movement. Repeat gently and carefully for a total of 10 breaths.

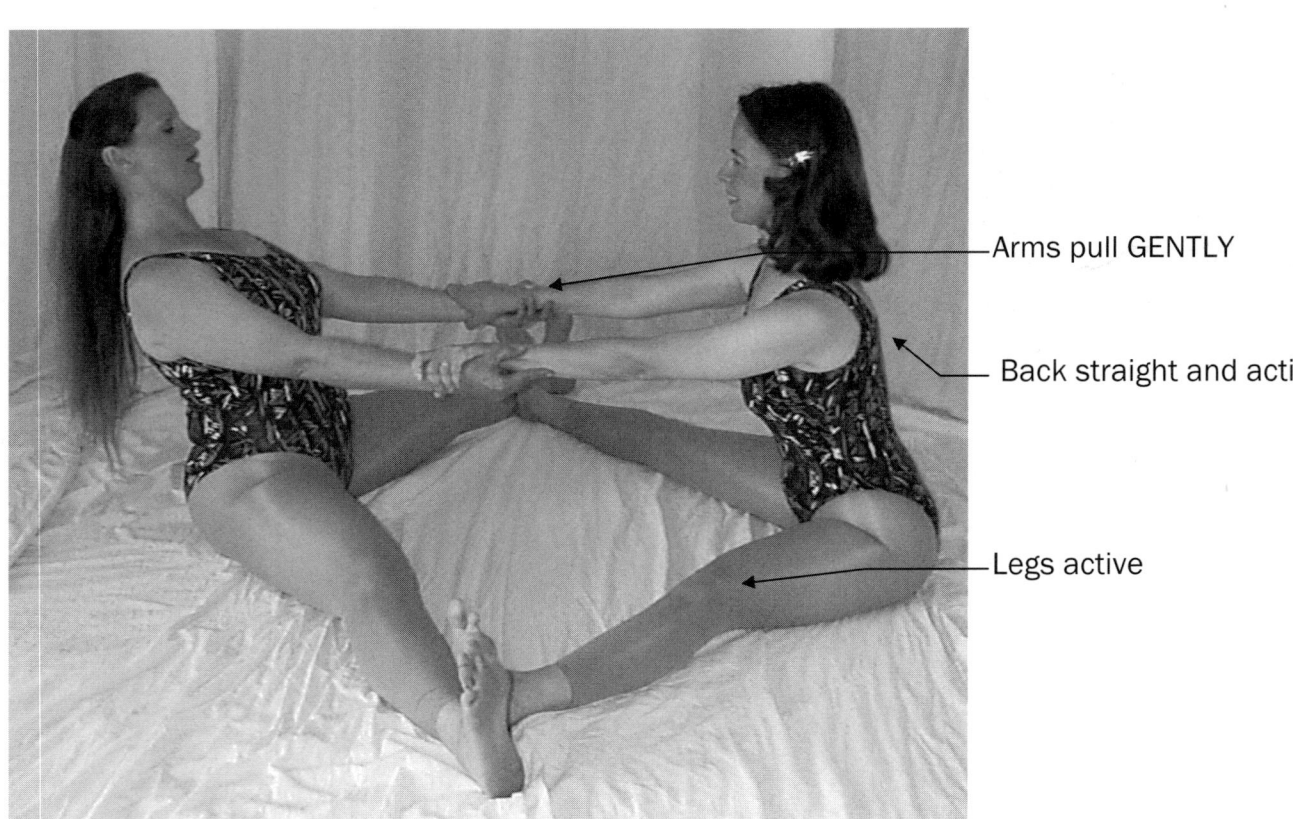

Arms pull GENTLY

Back straight and active

Legs active

Learning How to Give AND Receive.

Pyramid (Upavista Konasana 4)

All Levels

Caution - Do **NOT** pull yourself or your Partner any farther than is comfortable for your legs, back, and upper body.

Instructions
1. Start sitting face to face, feet to feet, with both Partners legs spread as wide as is comfortable for each. The LESS flexible Partner places the soles of their feet on the inside of the MORE flexible Partner's legs.
2. Both Partners EXHALE and lean into a forward bend as far as is comfortable until heads lightly touch and fhiger tips can touch toes.

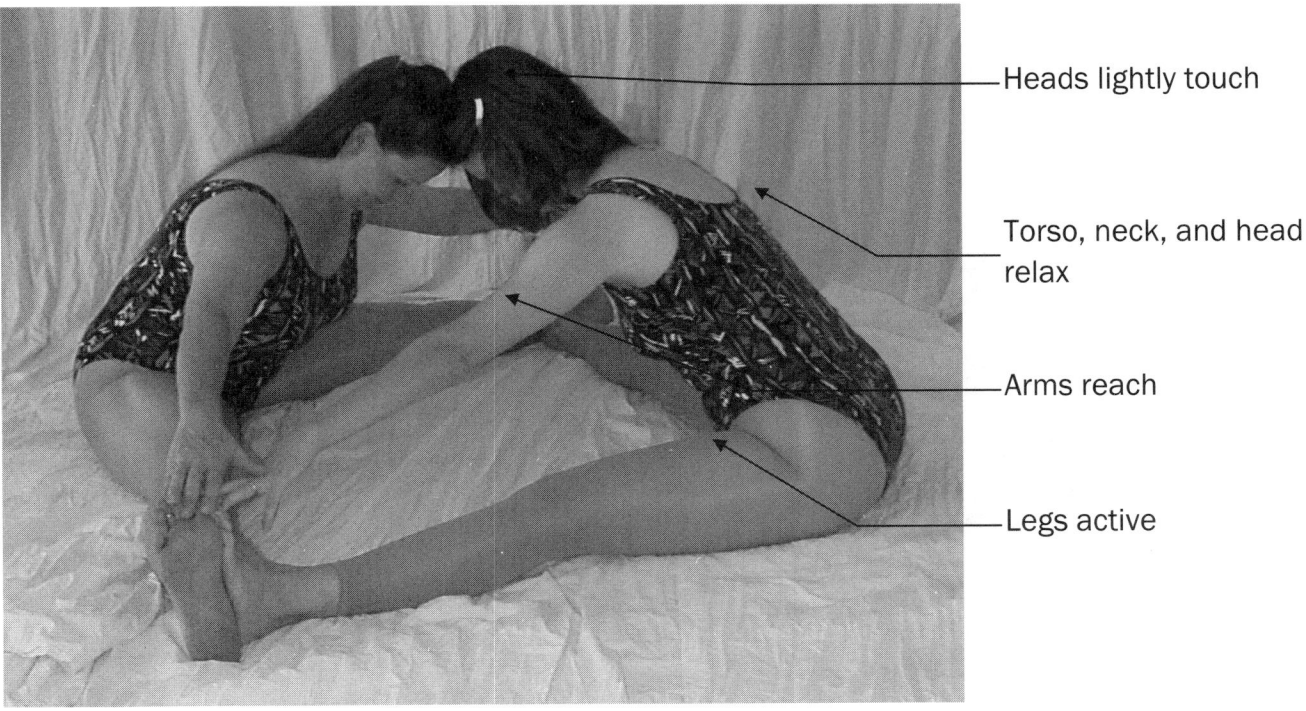

— Heads lightly touch

Torso, neck, and head relax

— Arms reach

— Legs active

Feel the power of the structure of a pyramid, the support, the strength.

Diamond (Upavista Konasana 5)

All Levels

Caution - Do **NOT** stretch yourself any farther than is comfortable for your legs, back, and upper bodies.

Instructions

1. Start sitting face to face, feet to feet, with both Partners legs spread as wide as is comfortable for each. The LESS flexible Partner places the soles of their feet on the inside of the MORE flexible Partner's legs.
2. Both Partners INHALE, stretch their arms over their head, and turn their torsos towards the RIGHT.
3. Both Partners EXHALE, lean forward from the hips, and reach towards their RIGHT foot.

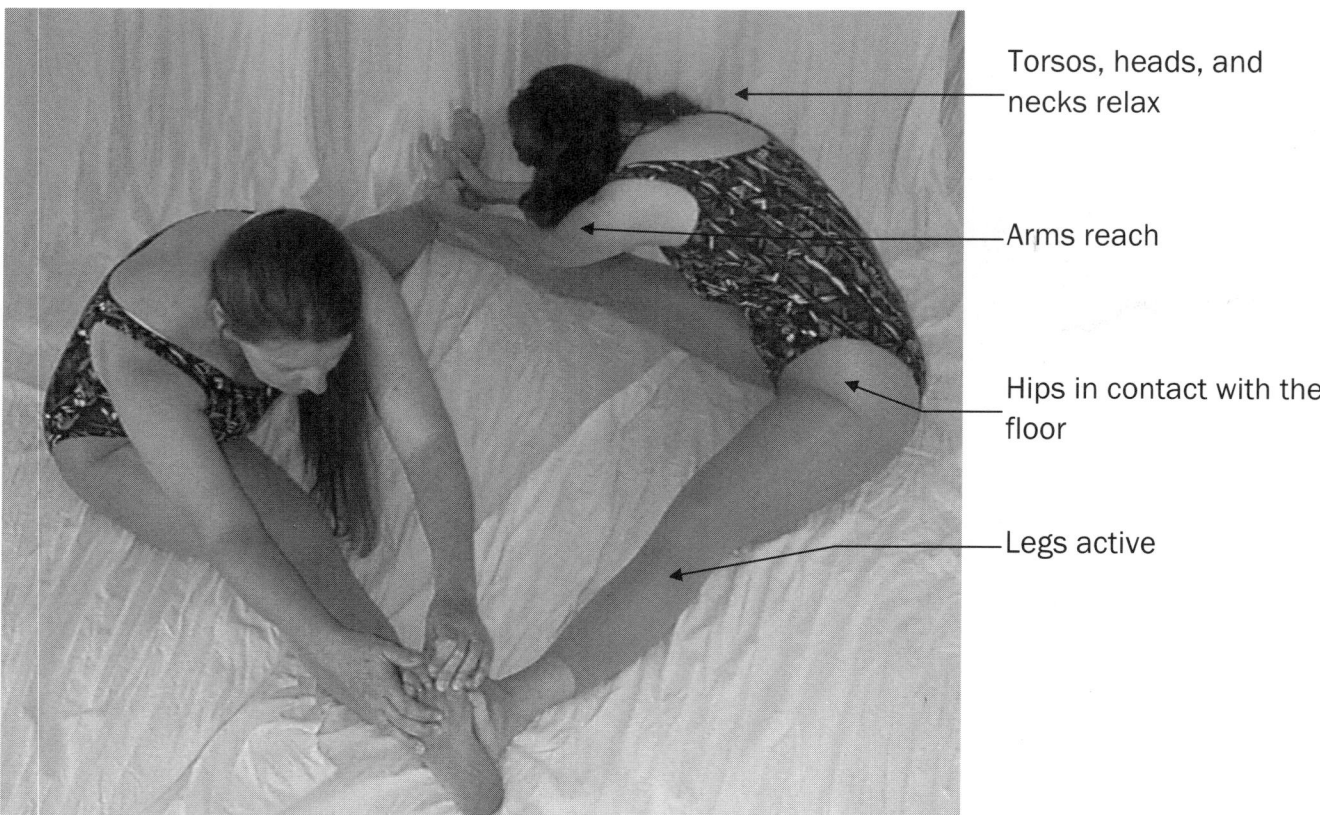

Torsos, heads, and necks relax

Arms reach

Hips in contact with the floor

Legs active

Go to the base of the pyramid to find the entrance.

Pinwheel (Parivrtta Upavista Konasana 1)

All Levels

Caution - Do **NOT** stretch yourself any farther than is comfortable for your legs, back, and upper bodies.

Instructions
1. Start sitting face to face, feet to feet, with both Partners legs spread as wide as is comfortable for each. The LESS flexible Partner places the soles of their feet on the inside of the MORE flexible Partner's legs.
2. Both Partners INHALE, stretch their LEFT arms over their head, and clasp hands, wrists, or forearms.
3. Both Partners EXHALE, twist to the LEFT, stretch their RIGHT hands towards their Partners' RIGHT foot.

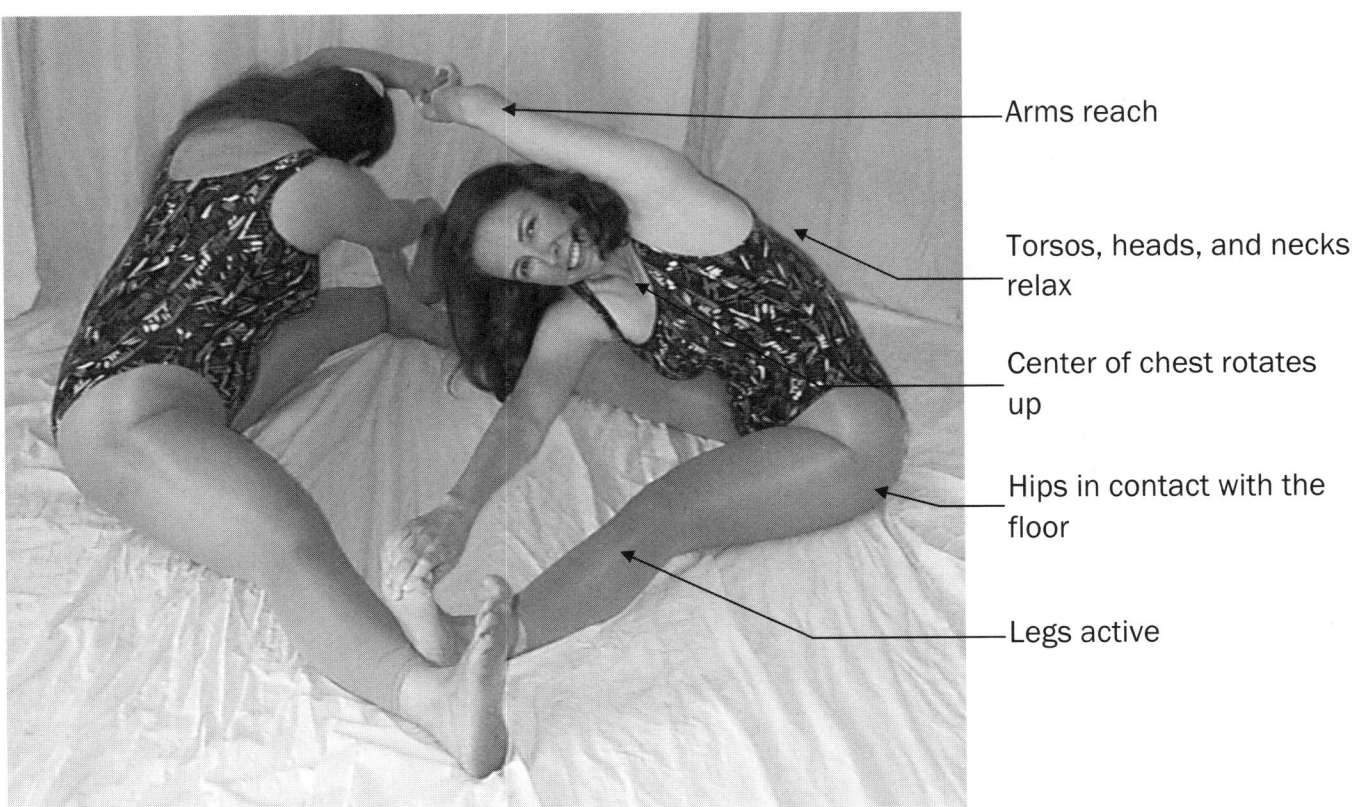

Arms reach

Torsos, heads, and necks relax

Center of chest rotates up

Hips in contact with the floor

Legs active

Go deep into the pyramid to find the treasure inside.

Dancing Pinwheel (Parivrtta Upavista Konasana 2)

All Levels

Caution - Do **NOT** stretch yourself any farther than is comfortable for your legs, back, and upper bodies.

Instructions
1. Start sitting face to face, feet to feet, with both Partners legs spread as wide as is comfortable for each. The LESS flexible Partner places the soles of their feet on the inside of the MORE flexible Partner's legs.
2. Partners clasp LEFT hands, wrists, or forearms.
3. Both Partners INHALE and stretch their RIGHT arms over their heads.
4. Both Partners EXHALE, stretch their torsos to the LEFT, and reach for their Partners' RIGHT feet with their RIGHT hands.

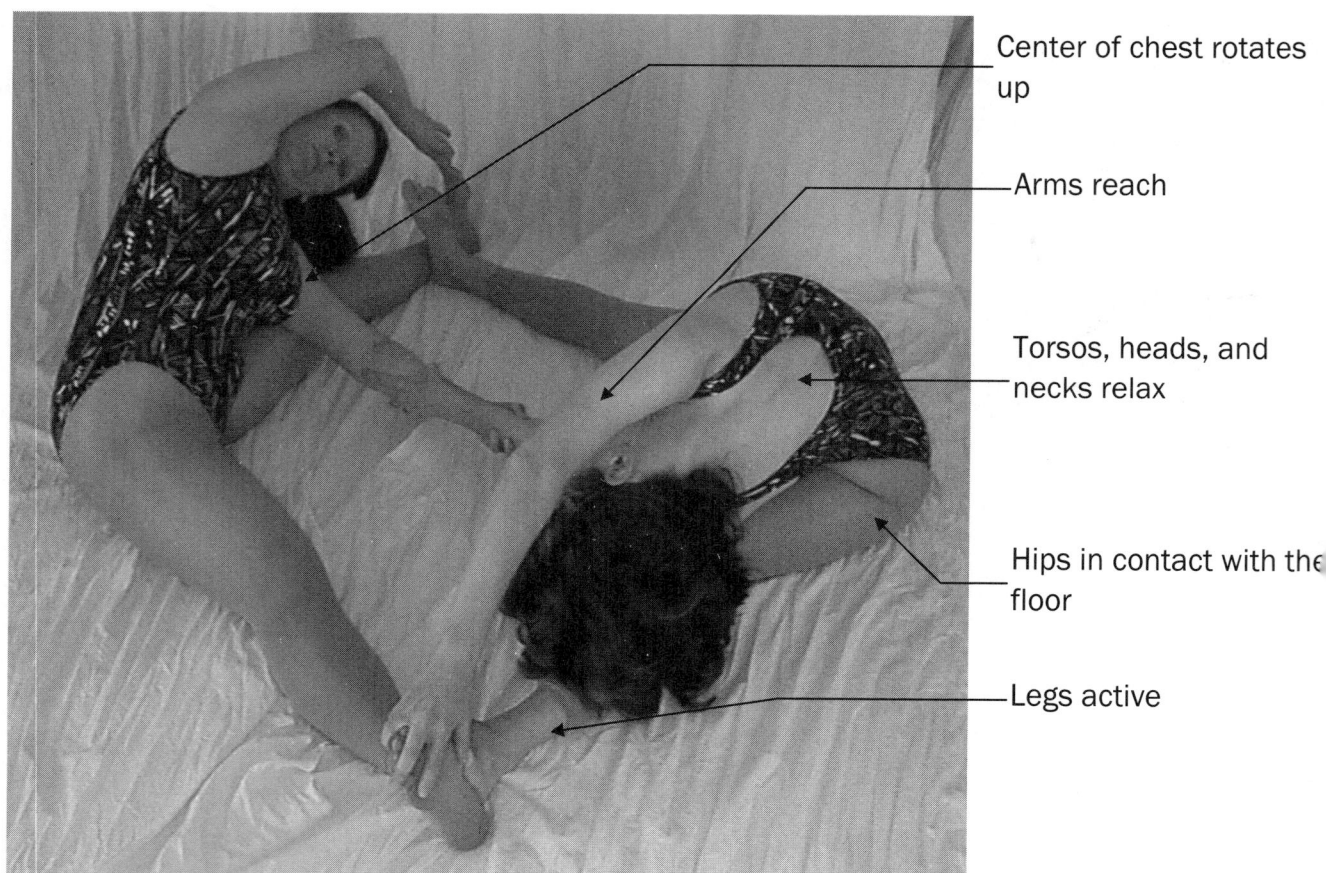

Center of chest rotates up

Arms reach

Torsos, heads, and necks relax

Hips in contact with the floor

Legs active

Hearts Ascending Upwards

Boat (Ardha Navasana)

Intermediate Level

Instructions

1. Start with Partners sitting in face to face on the floor with each Partners legs bent at the knees, the soles of their feet on the floor, and their toes touching. The exact distance between them will be determined by the length of their arms.
2. Clasp fingers as shown.
3. Raise legs and extend until straight.
4. Match feet.

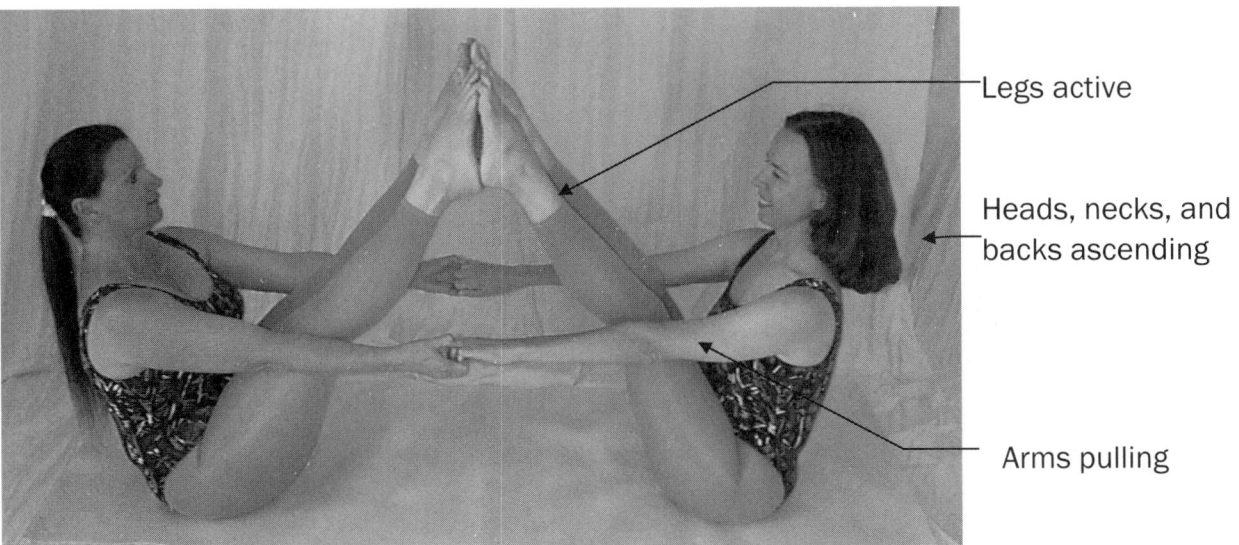

Legs active

Heads, necks, and backs ascending

Arms pulling

Obstacles to Connection

Head to Knee (Janu Sirsasana 1)

All Levels

Caution - Do **NOT** stretch any farther than is comfortable for your backs.

Instructions
1. Start with Partner 1 sitting on the floor with legs stretched out in front.
2. Partner 1 bends their LEFT leg at the knee and places the sole of the foot on the inside of their RIGHT thigh.
3. Partner 2 assumes the same position opposite Partner 1 and adjusts their position until the Partners' RIGHT feet touch the other Partners' LEFT shin as shown.
4. Both Partners INHALE, stretch their arms up and bend forward from the hips until their heads touch lightly and their arms rest on the other Partners' shoulders. Repeat on the other side.

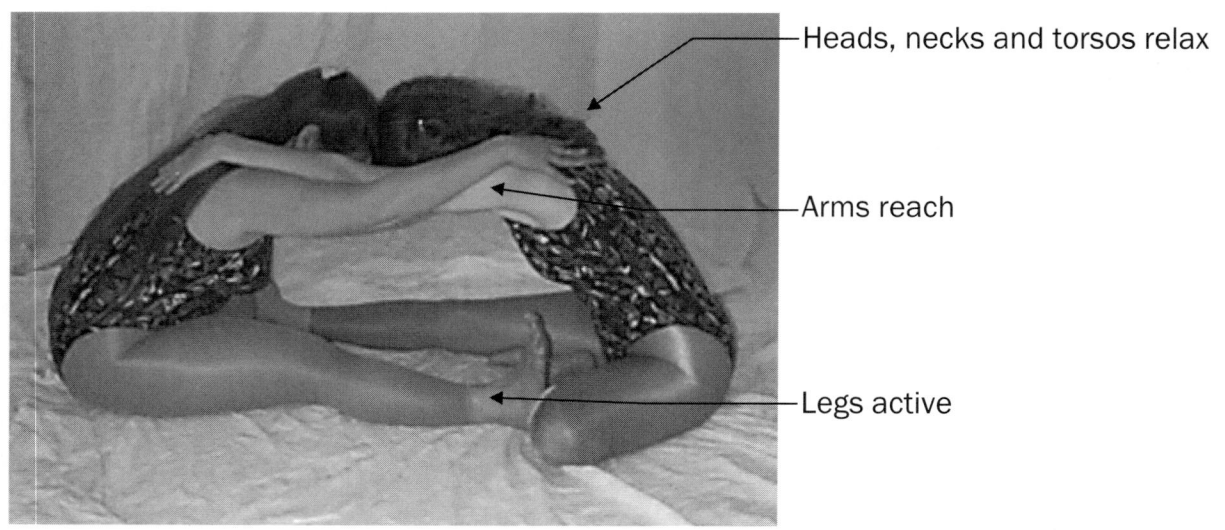

Heads, necks and torsos relax

Arms reach

Legs active

Surrender to Self

Half-Bound Forward Fold (Janu Sirsasana 2)

Intermediate/Advanced Levels

Caution - Do **NOT** stretch any farther than is comfortable.

Instructions
1. Start with Partner 1 sitting on the floor with legs stretched out in front. Partner 1 bends their LEFT leg at the knee and places the sole of their foot on the inside of their RIGHT thigh.
2. Partner 2 assumes the same position opposite Partner 1 and adjusts their position until the Partners' LEFT shins touch.
3. Both Partners INHALE, stretch their arms up and bend forward from the hips as far as is comfortable.
4. Partners' INSIDE arms reach across their Partners' lower back and Partners' OUTSIDE arms reach back and across to grasp their Partners' INSIDE arms. Repeat on the other side.

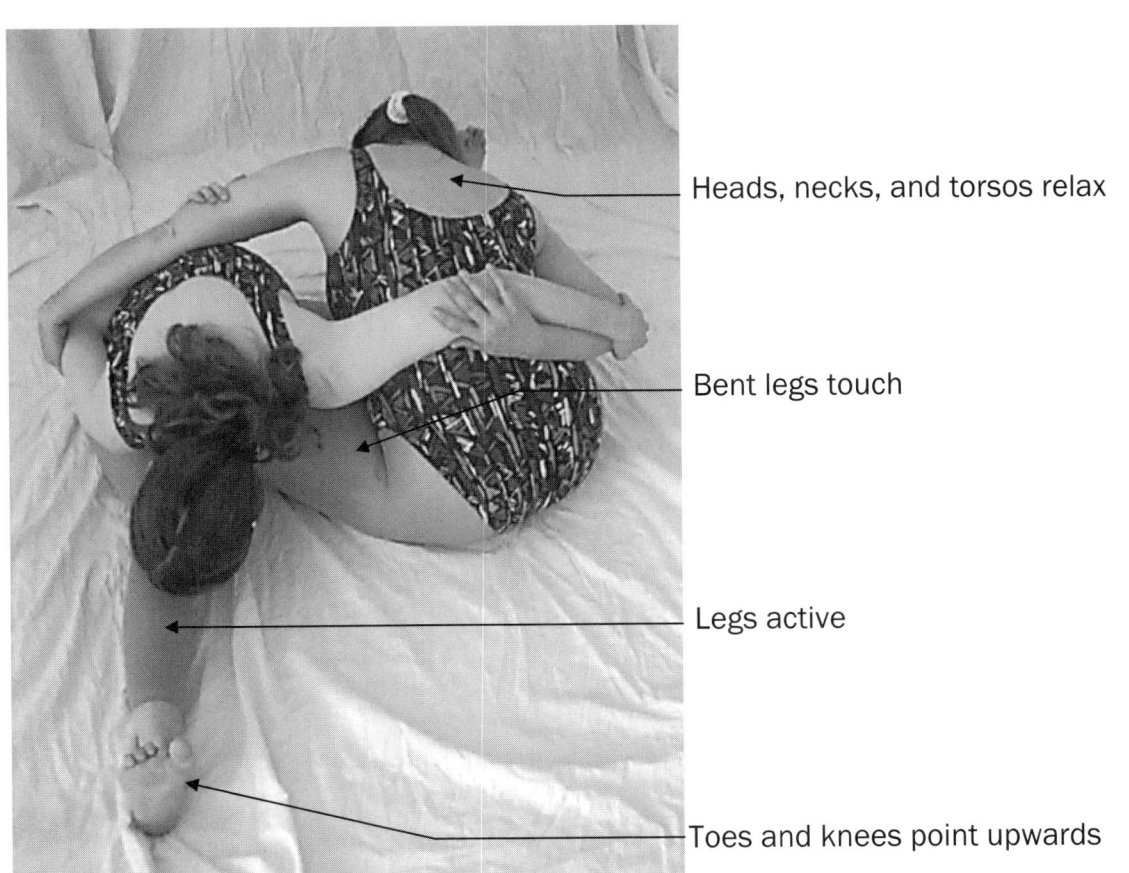

Heads, necks, and torsos relax

Bent legs touch

Legs active

Toes and knees point upwards

Surrender to Other

Rolled Fold (Parivrtta Janu Sirsasana 1)

Intermediate/Advanced Levels

Caution - Do **NOT** stretch or twist any farther than is comfortable.

Instructions
1. Start with Partners sitting hip to hip and side by side on the floor with legs stretched out in front. Each Partner bends their OUTSIDE legs at the knees and places the sole of their foot on the inside of their INSIDE thigh. Their hips and straight legs should touch.
2. Both Partners INHALE, stretch their arms up and bend forward from the hips as far as is comfortable or until they touch their toes.
3. Partners twist their torsos towards the OUTSIDE and their OUTSIDE arms stretch upwards and touch palm to palm.
4. Partners' INSIDE arms reach across and grasp their Partners' leg or foot. Repeat on the other side.

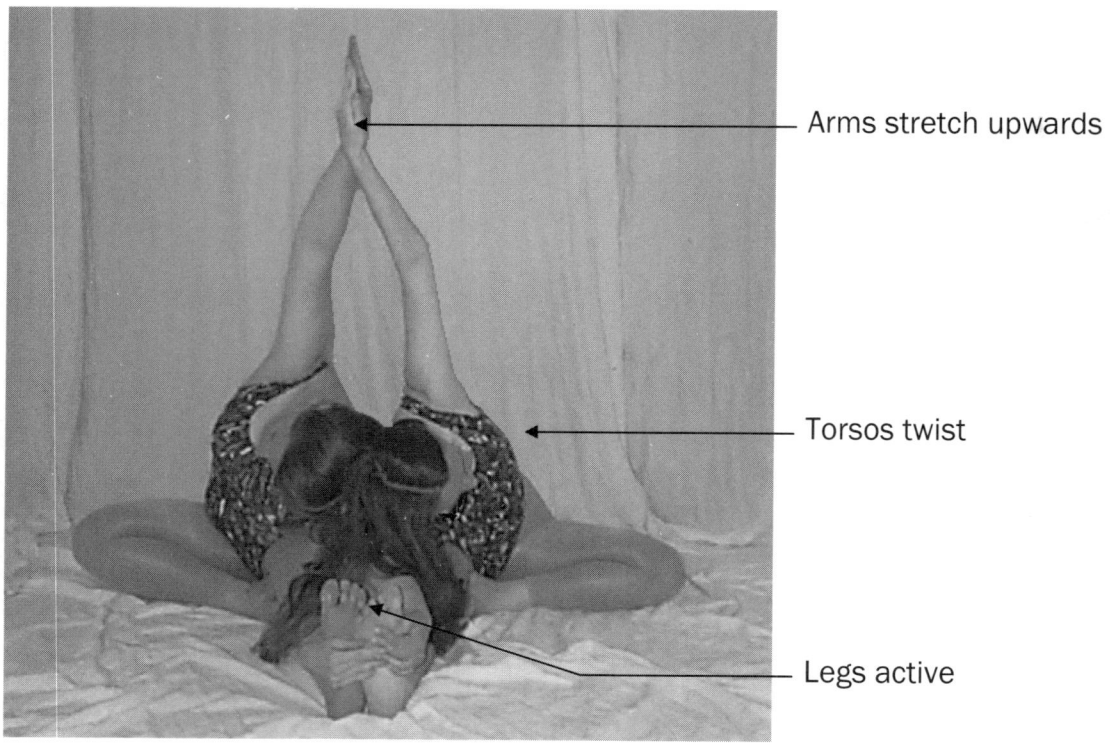

Arms stretch upwards

Torsos twist

Legs active

Surrender to Life

Starship (Parivrtta Janu Sirsasana 2)

Intermediate/Advanced Levels

Caution - Do **NOT** stretch or twist any farther than is comfortable.

Instructions
1. Start with Partners sitting side by side and 3-4' apart (exact distance depends on the length of their thighs) on the floor with legs stretched out in front. Each Partner bends their INSIDE legs at the knees and places the sole of their foot on the inside of their INSIDE thigh. Their knees should touch.
2. Both Partners INHALE, stretch their arms up and bend forward from the hips as far as is comfortable or until they touch their toes.
3. Partners twist their torsos towards the INSIDE and their INSIDE arms stretch upwards and over their heads to touch their own toes.
4. Partners' OUTSIDE arms reach across and grasp their Partners' wrists or forearms. Repeat on the other side.

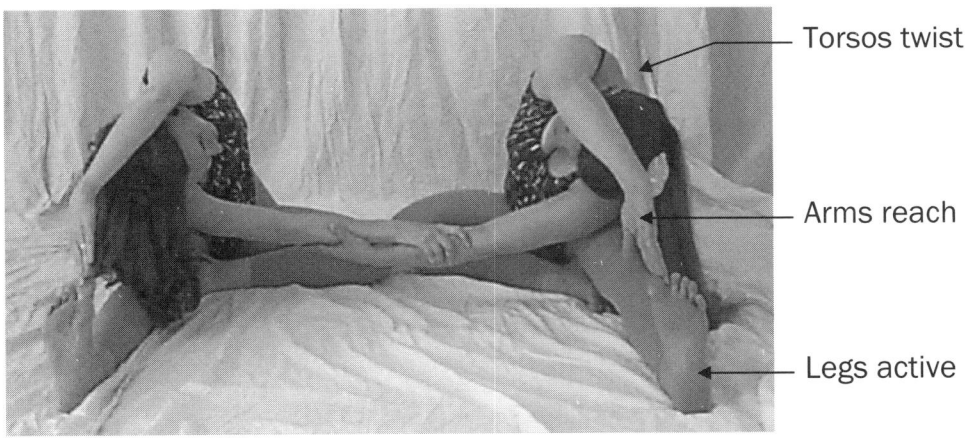

Torsos twist

Arms reach

Legs active

Surrender to Dharma

Forward Fold (Paschimottanasana)

Intermediate/Advanced Levels

Caution - Do **NOT** stretch any farther than is comfortable.

Instructions
1. Start with Partner 1 sitting on the floor with legs stretched out in front.
2. Partner 2 assumes the same position opposite Partner 1 and adjusts their position until the soles of the Partners' feet touch.
3. Both Partners INHALE, stretch their arms up and bend forward from the hips as far as is comfortable.
4. Partners' arms reach forward to grasp their Partners' hands, wrists, or forearms.

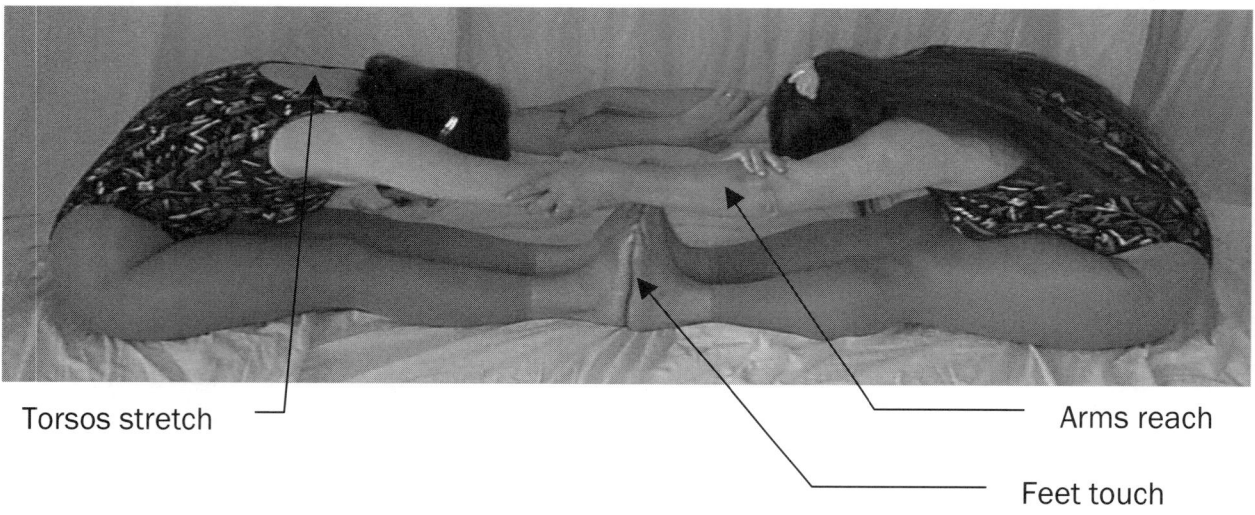

Torsos stretch

Arms reach

Feet touch

Surrender to your Higher Self

Other Forward Bends

The following is a list of poses where at least one Partner is bending forward during the pose or during one part of the pose:

BACKBENDS

&

COMBINATION POSES

Supported Rainbow (Chakrasana & Apanasana)

All Levels

Instructions

1. Start with Partner 1 lying on the floor on their back with their feet on Partner 2's gluteals and arms prepared to support Partner 1's shoulder blades.

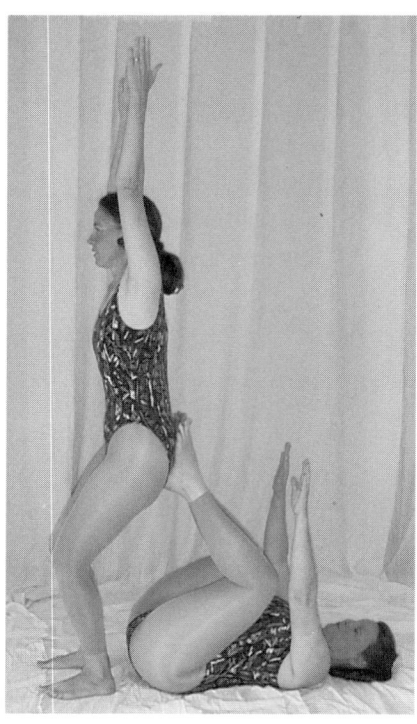

2. Partner 1 supports Partner 2's hips as Partner 2 raises hands up over head and moves into a backbend.

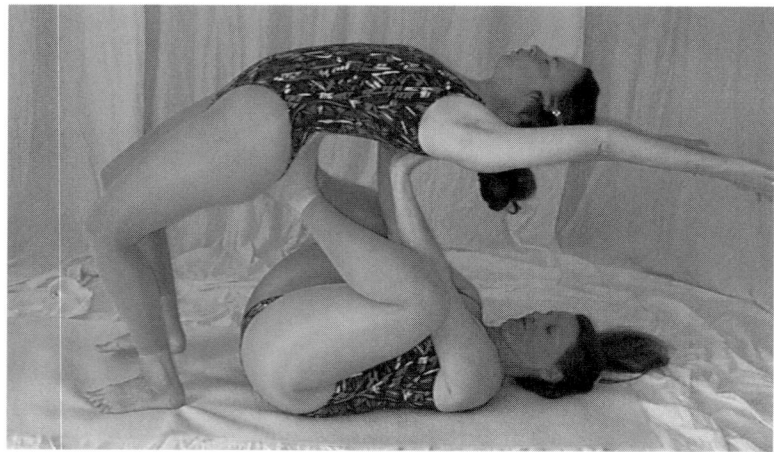

3. Partner 1 reaches out to support Partner 2's shoulder blades.
4. Partner 1 helps lower Partner 2 into the backbend until Partner 2's hands are firmly supporting them on the floor behind Partner 1's shoulders.

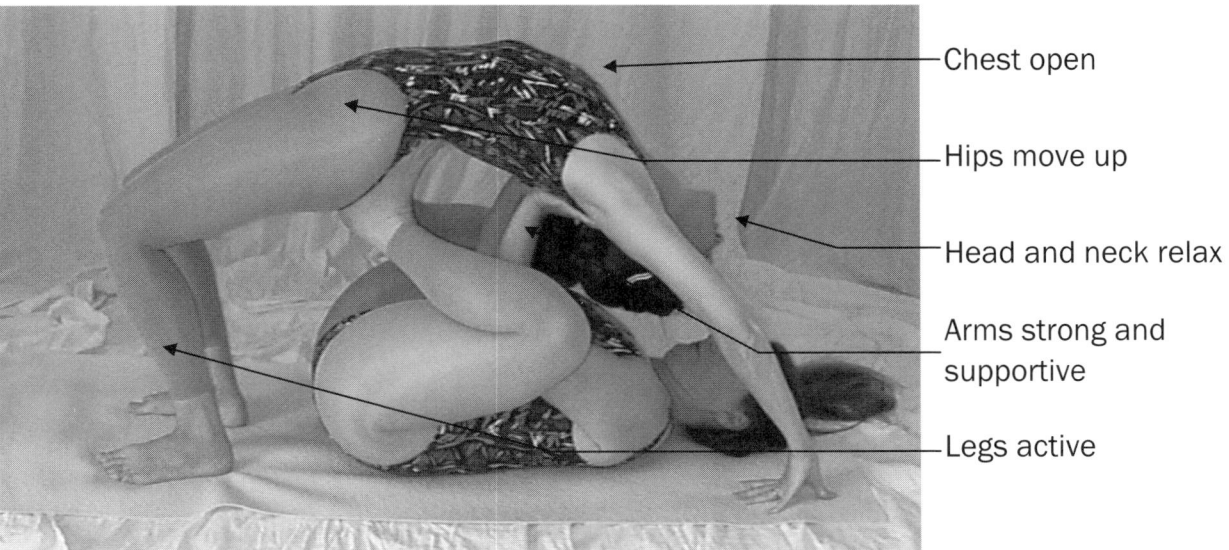

Chest open

Hips move up

Head and neck relax

Arms strong and supportive

Legs active

Laugh, Giggle

Note: to come out of this pose, Partner 1 pushes Partner 2 up with arms and legs.

Arm-Supported Backbend & Forward Pull Vinyasa (Figurehead Pose, Uttanasana, & Virbhadrasana II)

All Levels

Caution - Do not stretch your Partner's back any farther than is comfortable for them.

Instructions
1. Start with Partner 1 standing facing sideways and Partner 2 with legs 3-4 1/2' apart facing forward. Partner 2's RIGHT foot should be touching Partner 1,s heels.
2. Partner 2 turns LEFT foot 90 degrees away form midline and the Partners clasp hands as shown.
3. Partner 1 moves forward keeping head and chest up (also called the "Figurehead Pose") while at the same time Partner 2 bends their LEFT leg at the knee as shown (also called the "Warrior II Pose").

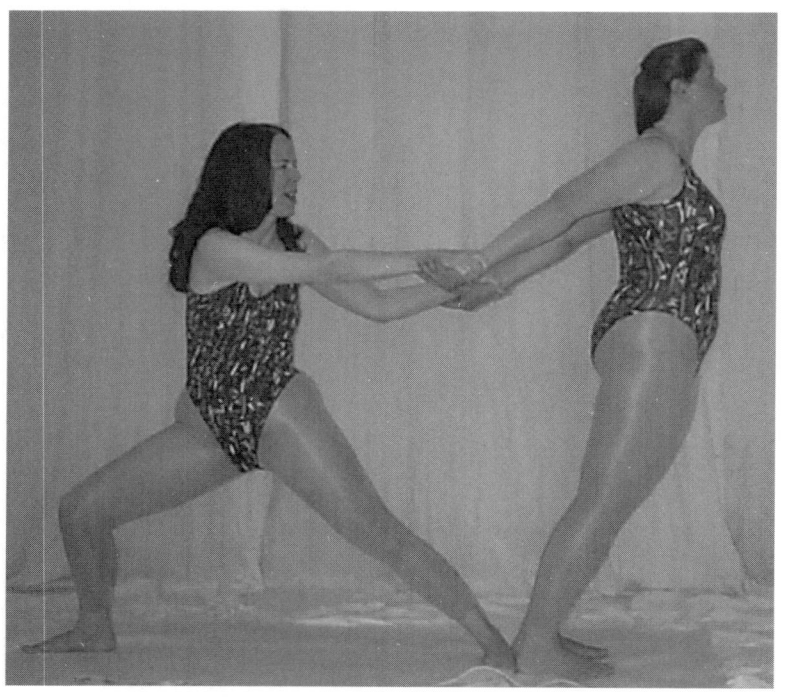

4. The Partners move back to the starting position then Partner 1 bends forward (also called the "Standing Forward Bend Pose") while at the same time Partner 2 moves back into the Warrior II Pose.

5. Repeat the movements as long as they are comfortable or up to 10 times.

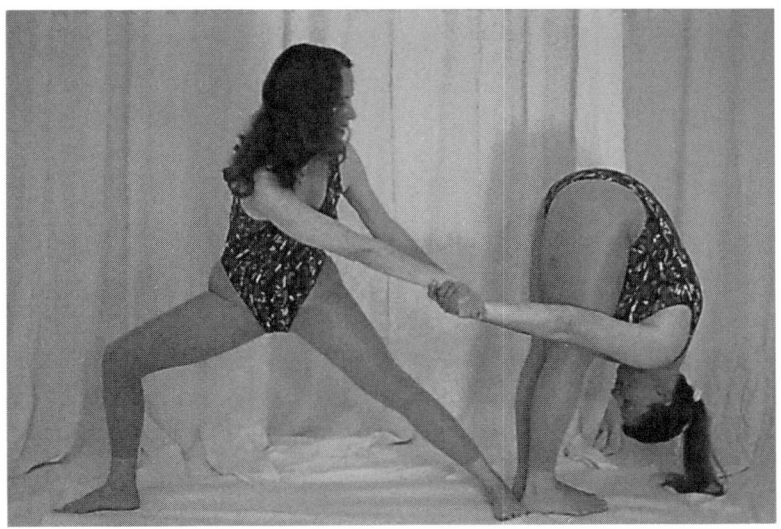

Ebb and Flow with the Breath

Note: Partner 2 should always be either standing or in the Warrior II Pose, never bent over as shown below.

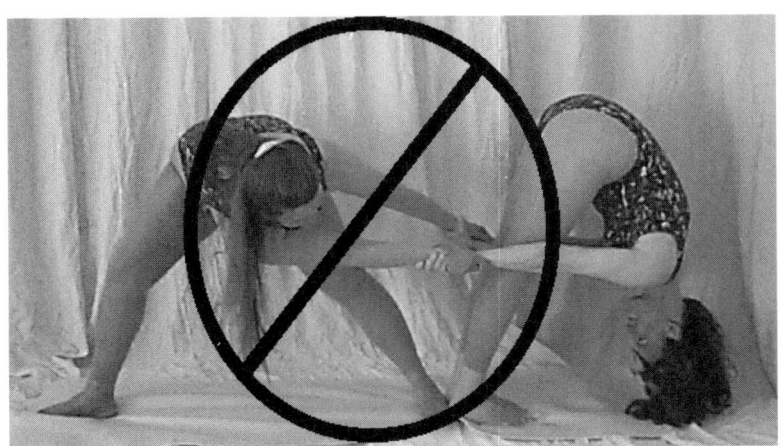

Back Stretcher (Utkatasana & Sitting Backbend)

All Levels

Caution - Do not stretch your Partner's back any farther than is comfortable for them.

Instructions
1. Start with Partner 1 sitting on the floor with legs stretched out in front.
2. Partner 2 stands behind Partner 1 with their feet approximately the same width as Partner 1's mid-back (the exact distance between the Partners will have to be adjusted depending on the height and build of each Partner).
3. Partner 2 bends their legs at the knees until they touch Partner 1's mid-back while at the same time Partner 1 stretches their arms overhead to clasp Partner 2's shoulders or neck as shown.
4. Partner 2 places their hands on Partner 1's armpits and GENTLY pulls them back while at the same time pressing their knees into Partner 1's mid-back

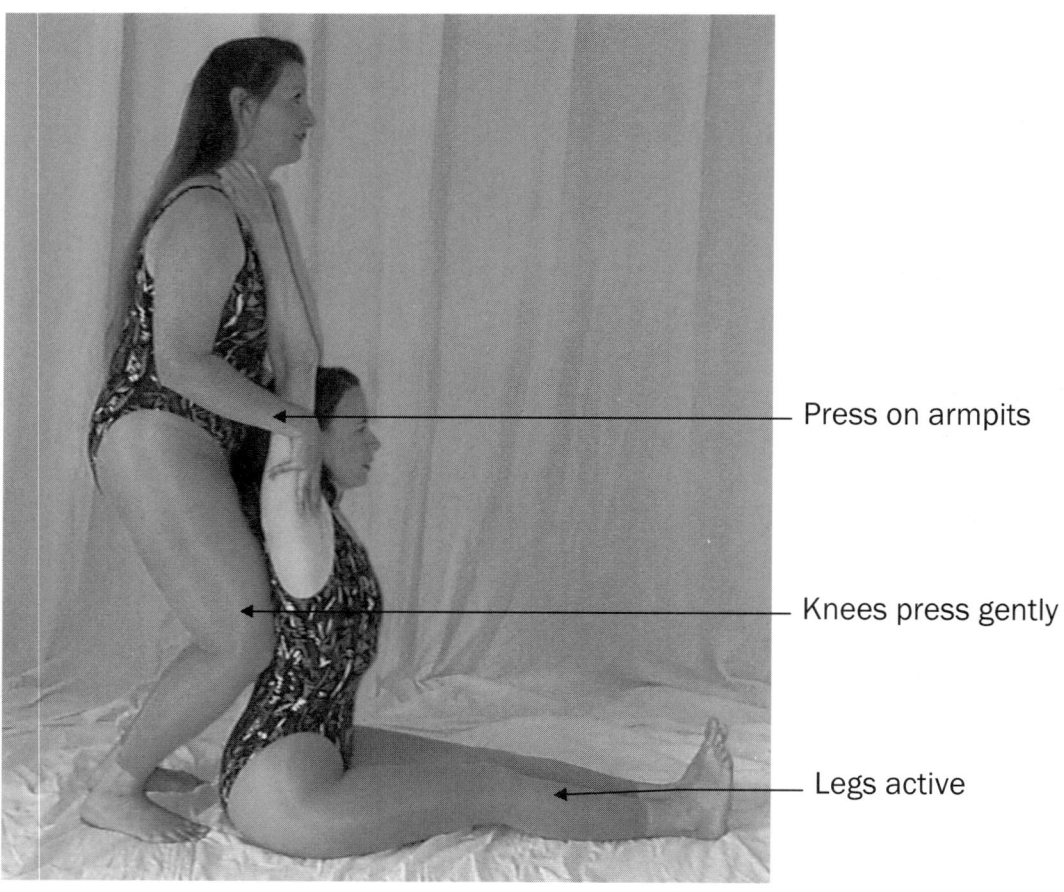

Press on armpits

Knees press gently

Legs active

Ohhhhhhhhh

Stretched Cobra (Bujangasana 1)

All Levels

Instructions
1. Start with Partner 1 lying face down on the floor and Partner 2 squatting toe to toe at Partner 1's feet.
2. Partner 2 should adjust their squatting position according to Partner 1's back's flexibility; i.e. the Partners' toes touching if Partner 1's back is not very flexible, the Partners' toes slightly apart if Partner 1's back is more flexible than average, etc.).
3. Partner 2 wraps their hands around Partner 1's ankles and grips firmly. Partner 1 should not lift Partner 1's ankles. To insure they do not Partner 2 can place their index finger on the floor and make certain in stays there during the pose.
4. Partner 1 lifts their head, shoulders, and upper torso shown (also called a "Beginning" Cobra Pose) while Partner 2 supports and VERY GENTLY pulls on Partner 1's legs.

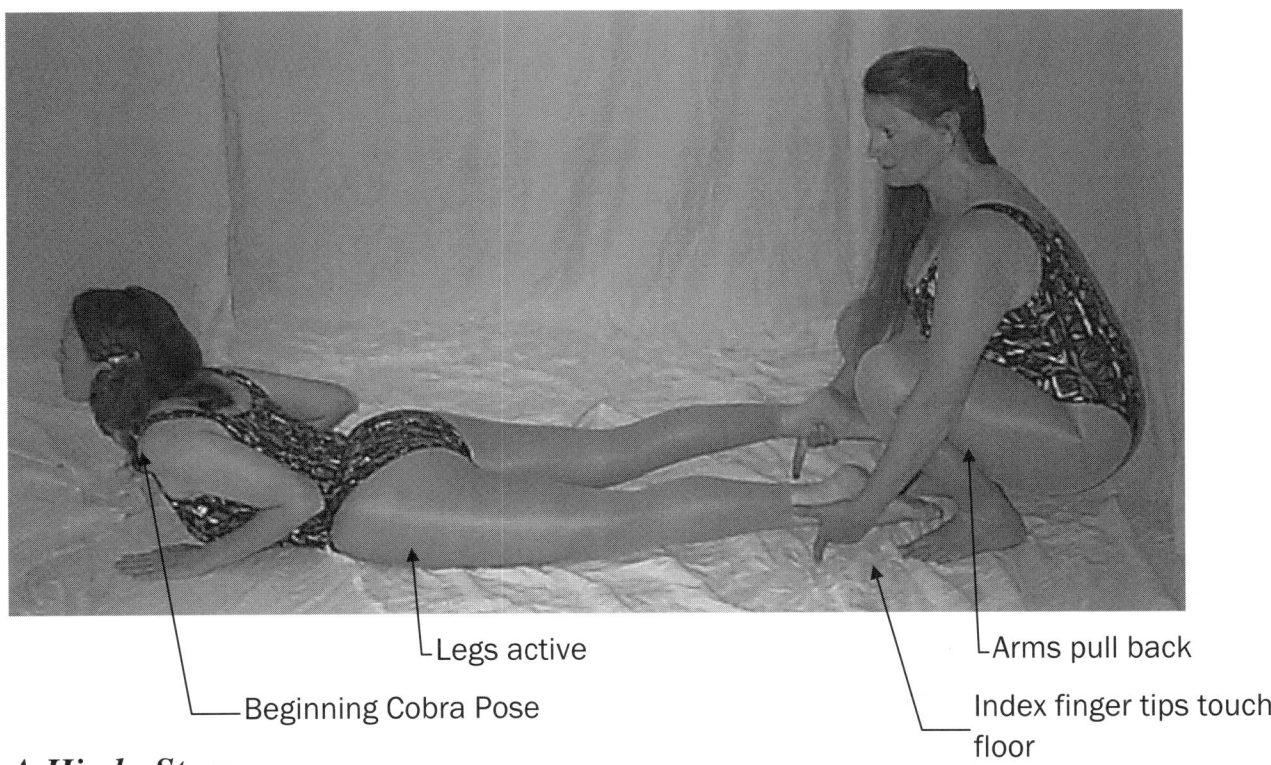

Legs active

Beginning Cobra Pose

Arms pull back

Index finger tips touch floor

A Hindu Story
Once a cobra went to a saint and said, "I want to be a good snake and attain liberation in this lifetime. Please, tell me what to do."
The saint said . . .

Supported Cobra (Bujangasana 2)

All Levels

Instructions

1. Start with Partner 1 lying on their stomach on the floor, arms out to the side and Partner 2 squatting with their feet on either side of Partner 1's waist.
2. Partner 2 sits down LIGHTLY on Partner 1's LOWER BACK. Partner 2's legs should be active and pushing at all times and their full weight should never be on Partner 1's back. Partner 1 STRONGLY engages their hip and leg muscles (this should be so strong Partner 2 can feel the movement). Partner 2 slides their hips back until they are sitting LIGHTLY on Partner 1's sacrum.

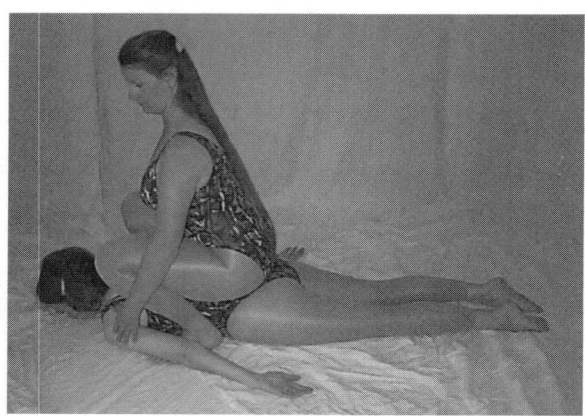

3. Partner 1 stretches their arms out into a "T". Partner 2 puts their hands through Partner 1's armpits and up around the shoulders until they see their fingers.
4. Partner 2 lifts (using strength in legs and arms, NOT lower back) into a supported Cobra Pose.

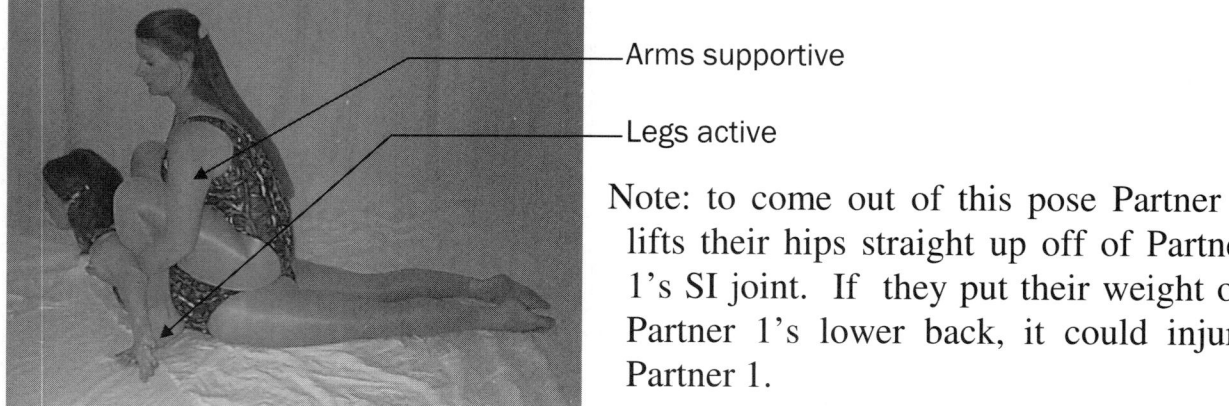

Arms supportive

Legs active

Note: to come out of this pose Partner 2 lifts their hips straight up off of Partner 1's SI joint. If they put their weight on Partner 1's lower back, it could injure Partner 1.

The saint said, "Love everyone and don't bite them."

Super Cobra (Bujangasana 3)

All Levels

Instructions

1. Follow steps 1 and 2 on previous page for "Supported Cobra."

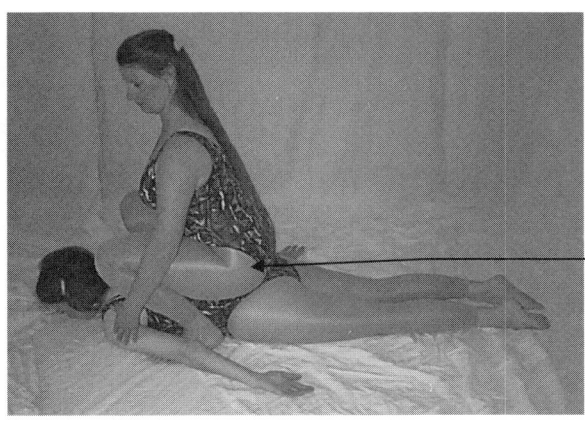

Hips rest very lightly on back

2. Partner 1 stretches their arms straight up over their head. Partner 2 puts their hands through Partner 1's armpits and up around the shoulders until they can see their fingers.
3. Partner 2 lifts (using strength in legs and arms, NOT lower back) into a supported Cobra Pose.

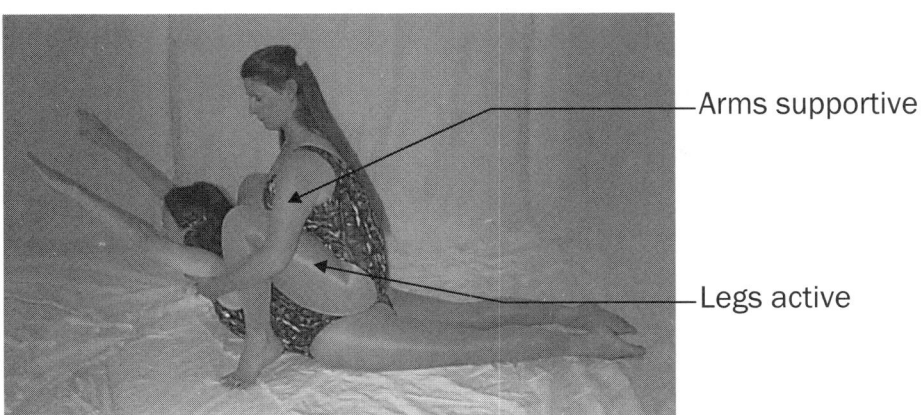

Arms supportive

Legs active

Note: To come out of this pose Partner lifts their hips straight up off of Partner 1's SI joint. If they put their weight on Partner 1's lower back, Partner 1could be injured.

The snake left and tried VERY hard to love everyone. However, he had been so fierce and wicked before, no one believed him. People beat him, threw stones at him, and tried to kill him, so he was forced to flee for his life back to the saint.

Flying Cobra (Bujangasana 4)

Advanced Level

Caution - This pose requires great shoulder flexibility and a very strong lower back in the Partner doing the Cobra portion.

Instructions
1. Partner 1 lies on their stomach on the floor while Partner 2 stands straddling Partner 1's legs at the knees.
2. Partner 2 grasps Partner 1's forearms just above wrists and pulls Partner 1 into the Flying Cobra Pose.
3. At the end of this series of Cobra Poses do the Pressed Leaf Pose (page 99).

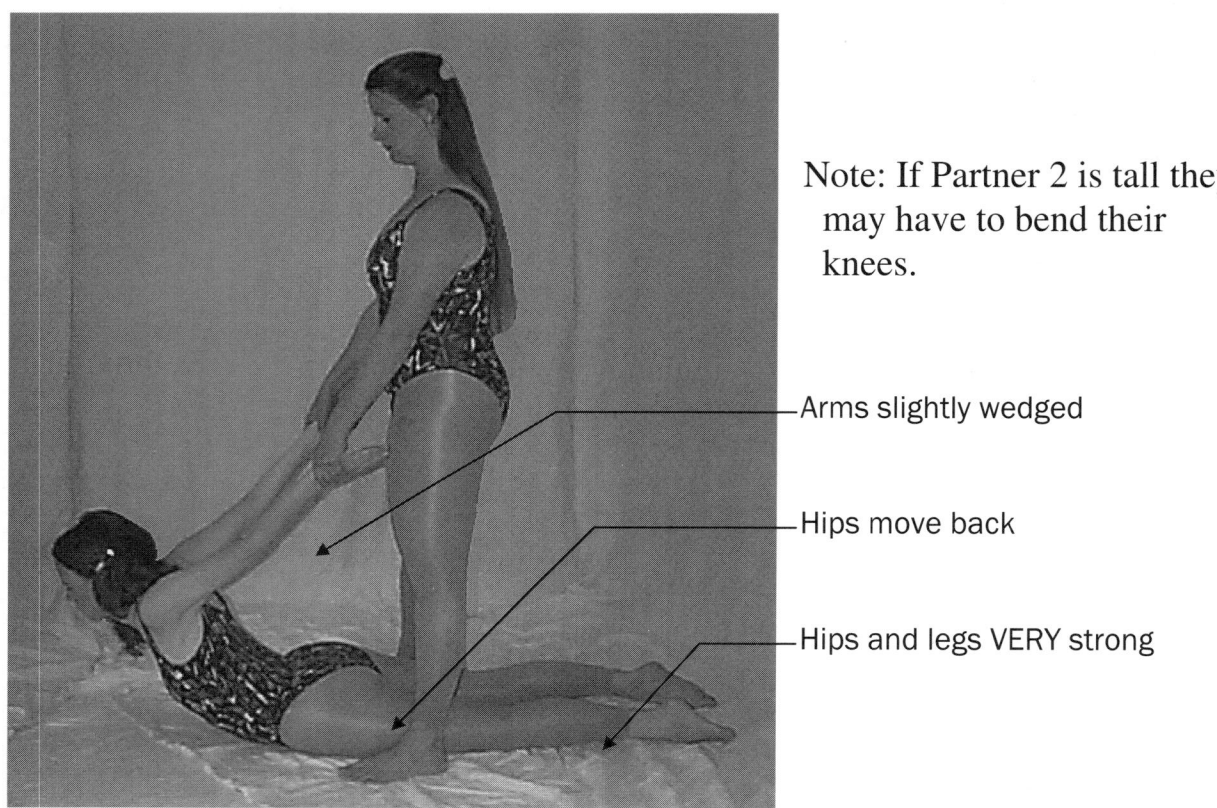

Note: If Partner 2 is tall they may have to bend their knees.

Arms slightly wedged

Hips move back

Hips and legs VERY strong

When the saint saw the broken and battered cobra he said, "Poor little snake. I didn't tell you couldn't hiss." The saint healed the snake and sent him back out into the world. The snake hissed at everyone he met and he coiled as if to strike. The people ran from him in terror. He loved everyone, he bit no one, and he achieved liberation in his lifetime.

Twisting Camel (Matsyendrasana & Ustrasana)

All Levels

Instructions
1. Partner 1 sits on floor with RIGHT leg stretched out in front and the LEFT leg bent at the knee with the sole of the LEFT foot on the floor.
2. Partner 2 kneels facing Partner 1's RIGHT hip.
3. Partners clasp wrists.
4. Partner 1 is gently pulled into a twist an Partner 2 moves into the Camel Pose.

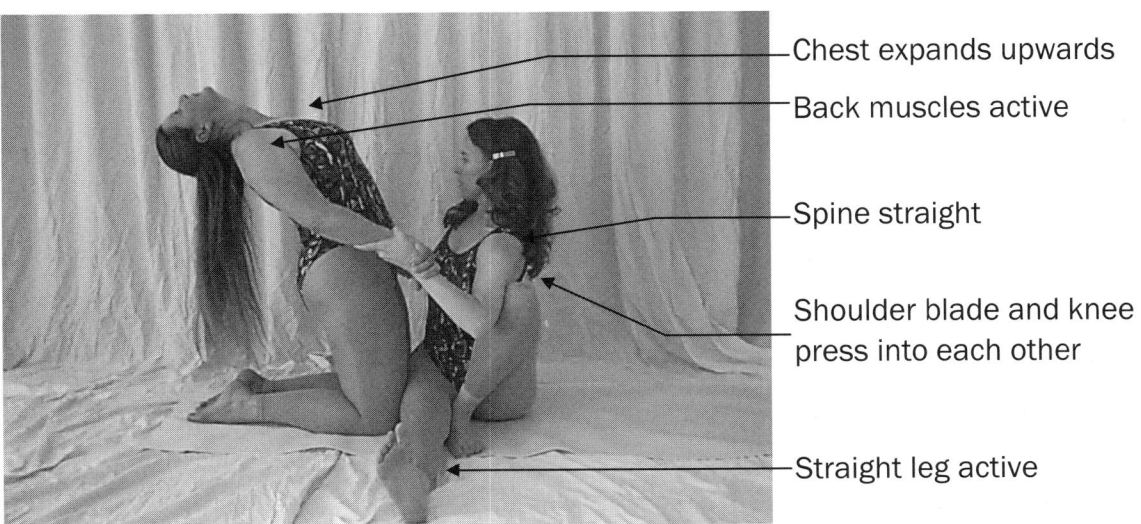

Chest expands upwards

Back muscles active

Spine straight

Shoulder blade and knee press into each other

Straight leg active

Watch the Lotus Open.

Putting on the Dog (Chakrasana & Adhomukha Svanasana)

All Levels

Instructions

1. Start with Partner 1 in position shown (also called "The Downward Facing Dog Pose").
2. Partner 2 straddles Partner 1's arms with legs bent at the knees.
3. Partner 2 matches upper hips to Partner 1's lower back, places hands beside hips, and pushes slightly with legs.
4. Partner 2 moves into backbend with arms at their sides (beginner), in a "T" (intermediate), or over their head (advanced).

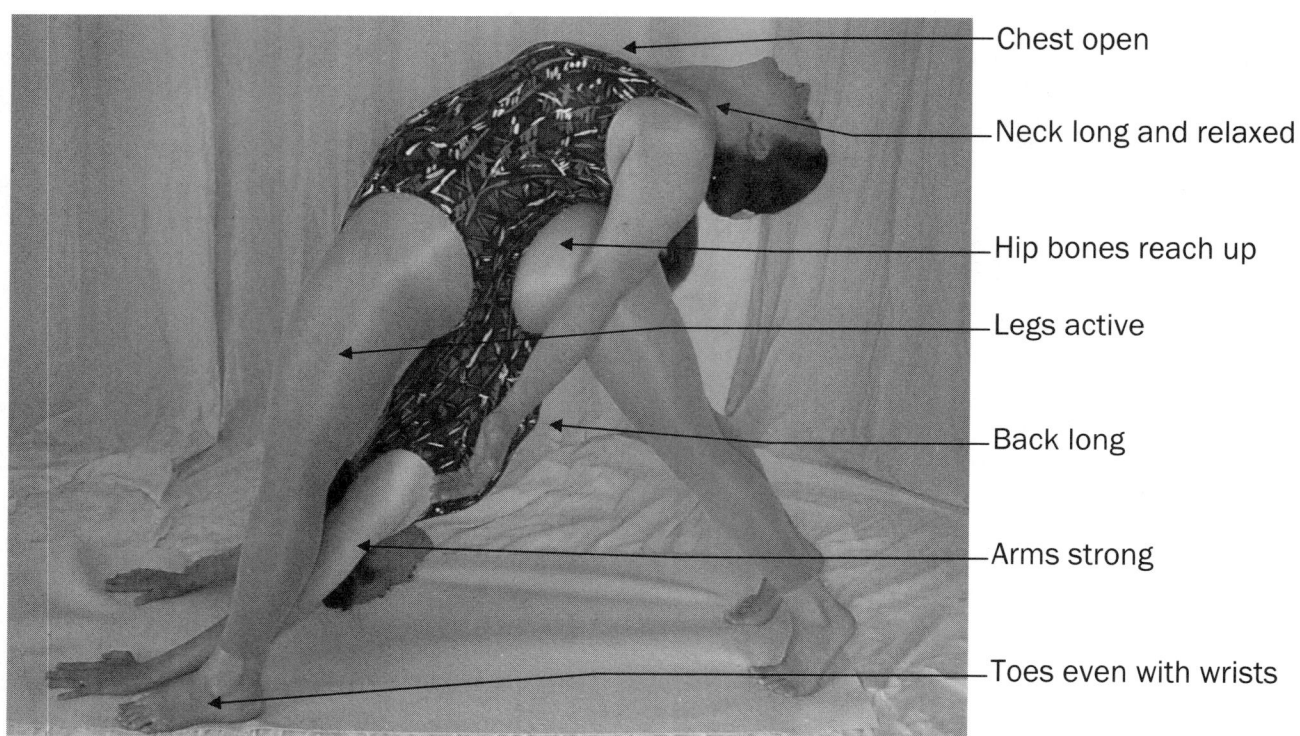

Support & Surrender

Tower of Power (Chakrasana & Uttanasana)

Intermediate Level

Instructions
1. Start with Partner 1 in a standing forward bend with hands on the floor for support.
2. Partner 2 stands 1- 2' behind Partner 1 facing away from them (the exact distance will depend on the height of the Partners).
3. Partner 2 matches their upper back to Partner 1's hips, places hands on top of Partner 1's hips, presses directly downwards with their hands, and engages legs.
4. Partner 2 moves into a backbend with arms reaching down. Partner 1 moves their arms into the position shown and Partner 2 lightly holds them as shown.

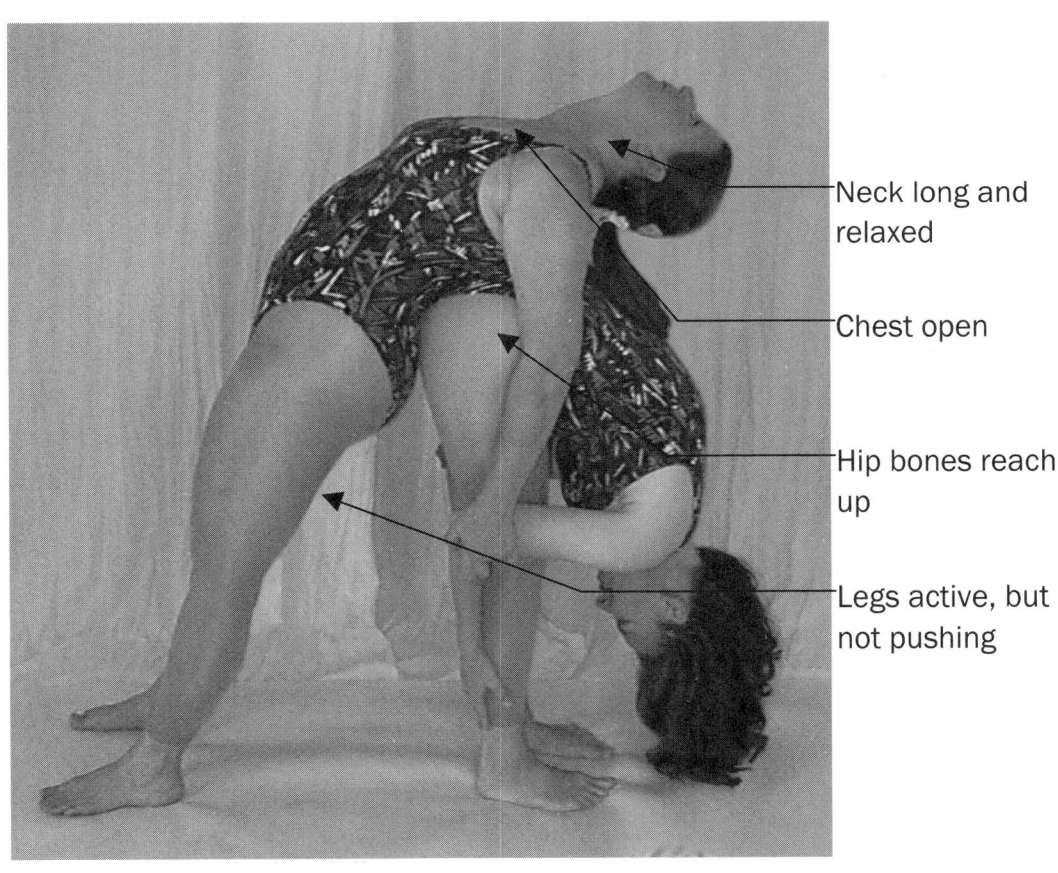

Neck long and relaxed

Chest open

Hip bones reach up

Legs active, but not pushing

Acceptance of Dharma

Hang the Yogi (Gajasana to Tadasana & Uttanasana)

Intermediate/Advanced Level

Cautions - See individual steps.

Instructions

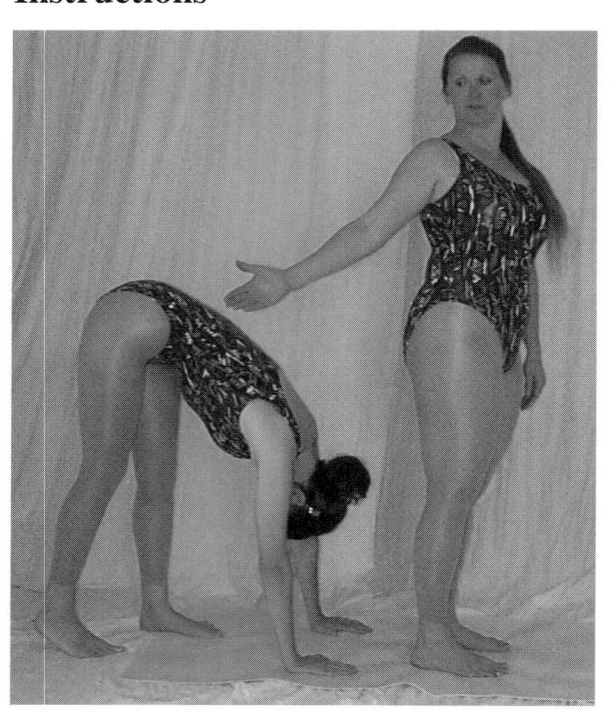

1. Start with Partner 1 standing and Partner 2 in position shown (also called "The Elephant Pose") behind Partner 1. Partner 1's head should be turned towards Partner 2's leading leg in preparation for Partner 2 to move into the Handstand.

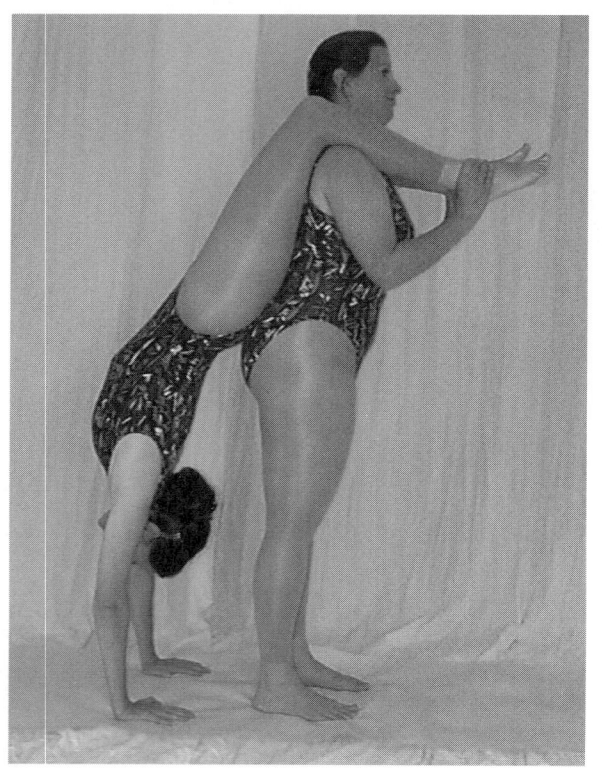

2. Partner 2 moves into Handstand with their legs resting lightly on the back of Partner 1's shoulders. Partner 1 moves in to Chair Pose (depth is dependent on Partner 2's height) until the back of Partner 2's knee joints can rest directly on top of Partner 1's shoulders. Partner 1 grips Partner 2's shins, pulls firmly straight outward and stands.

Caution - Do NOT pull lower legs down, pull out instead.

3. Partner 1 straightens knees and moves into a partial Standing Forward Bend lifting Partner 1 off the floor. Partner 2 grasps Partner 1's ankles/calves. Partners can remain in this part of the pose for up to 1 minute.

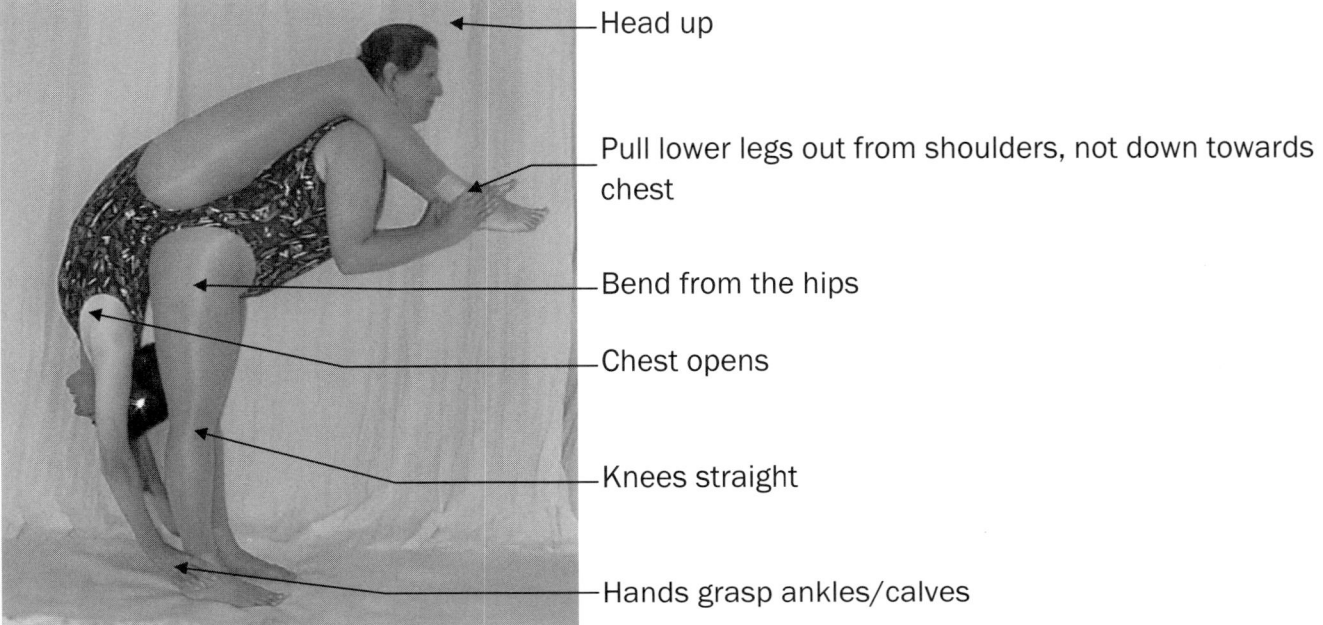

Head up

Pull lower legs out from shoulders, not down towards chest

Bend from the hips

Chest opens

Knees straight

Hands grasp ankles/calves

4. Partner 2 releases hands and Partner 1 moves farther into the Standing Forward Bend. Partners can remain in this part of the pose for up to 1 minute.

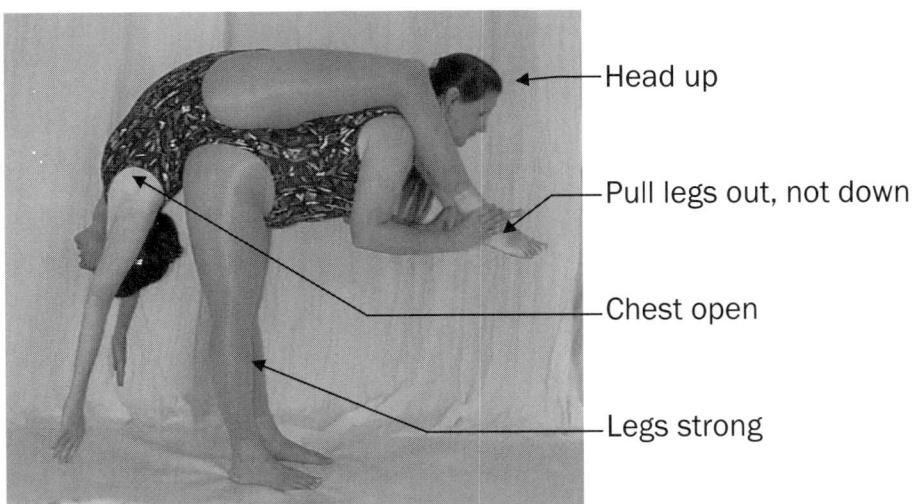

Head up

Pull legs out, not down

Chest open

Legs strong

5. Partner 2 LOWERS HEAD and completes Standing Forward Bend.

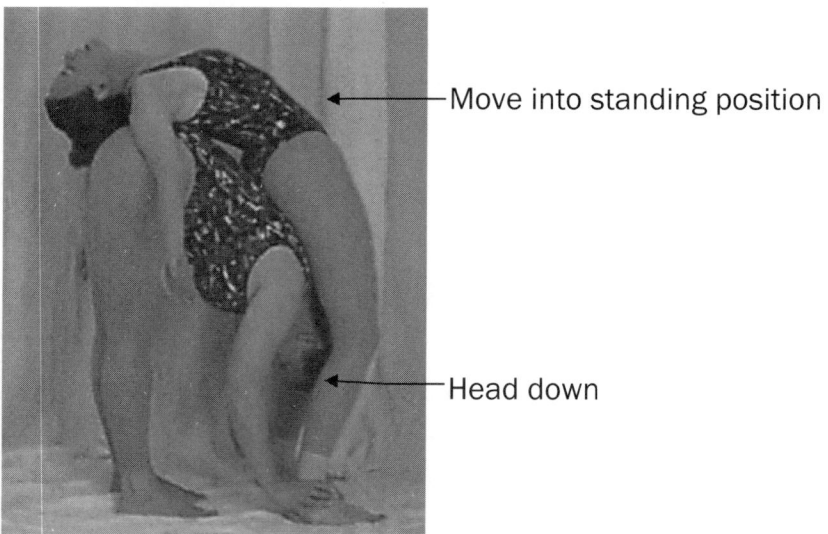

Move into standing position

Head down

6. Partner 1 moves to standing position.

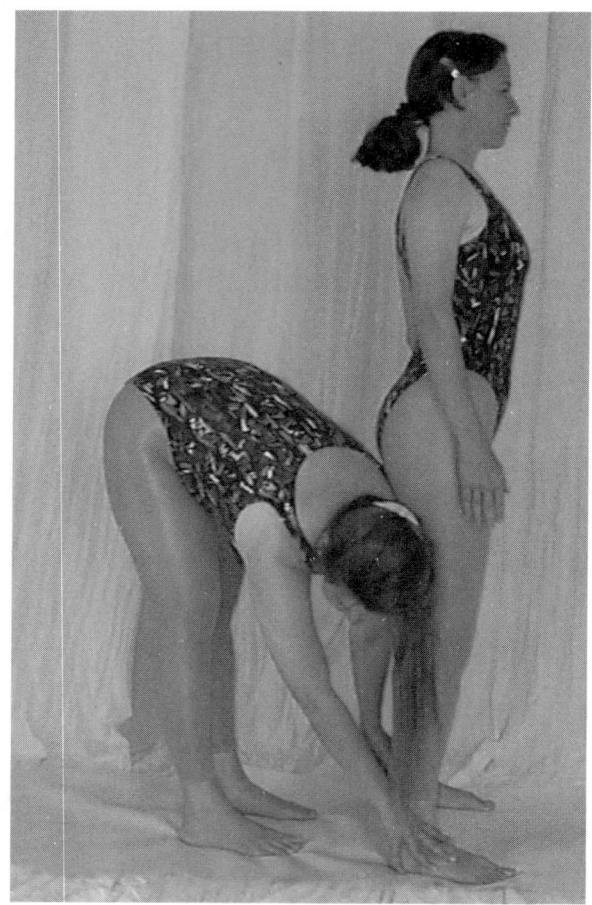

Trust

Other Backbends and Combination Poses

The following is a list of poses where at least one Partner is bending backward during the pose or during one part of the pose:

All Fish Poses - pages 49-55
Arm-Supported Backbend & Forward Pull Vinyasa (Figurehead Pose, Uttanasana, & Virbhadrasana II) - page 84
4Hang the Yoga for 3 or More (Uttanasana & Adhomukha Svasana to Tadasana) - page 121
Upward Facing Dog, Standing (Sama Adhomukha Svasana) – page 36

The following is a list of other combination poses:

All Fish Poses except pages 49-50
Hang the Yogi for 3 or More (Adhomukha Vrksasana to Chakrasana & Uttanasana for 3 or More) - page 121
Hip Lift (Savasana & Standing Squat) - page 107
Press & Release (Apanasana & Standing Squat) - page 106
Pressed Leaf (Balasana) - page 109
Pushing the Plough (Halasana) - page 111
Shoulderstand & Squat 1 (Sarvangasana & Squat 1) - page 43
Shoulderstand & Squat 2 (Sarvangasana & Squat 2) - page 44
Torso Lift (Savasana & Tadasana) - page 108
Watchtower (Savasana & a Sitting Pose) - page 115

TWISTS

Cheek to Cheek Comet (Parivrtta Janu Sirsasana 3)

All Levels

Instructions
1. Start sitting hip to hip, facing the same direction, legs stretched out in front.
2. Bend the OUTSIDE legs at the knees and bring the soles of the feet to rest somewhere comfortable on the inside edges of the thighs.
3. Turn towards INSIDE legs and use OUTSIDE arms to grasp inside edge of Partners' foot or leg.
4. Clasp INSIDE hands and stretch out arms.

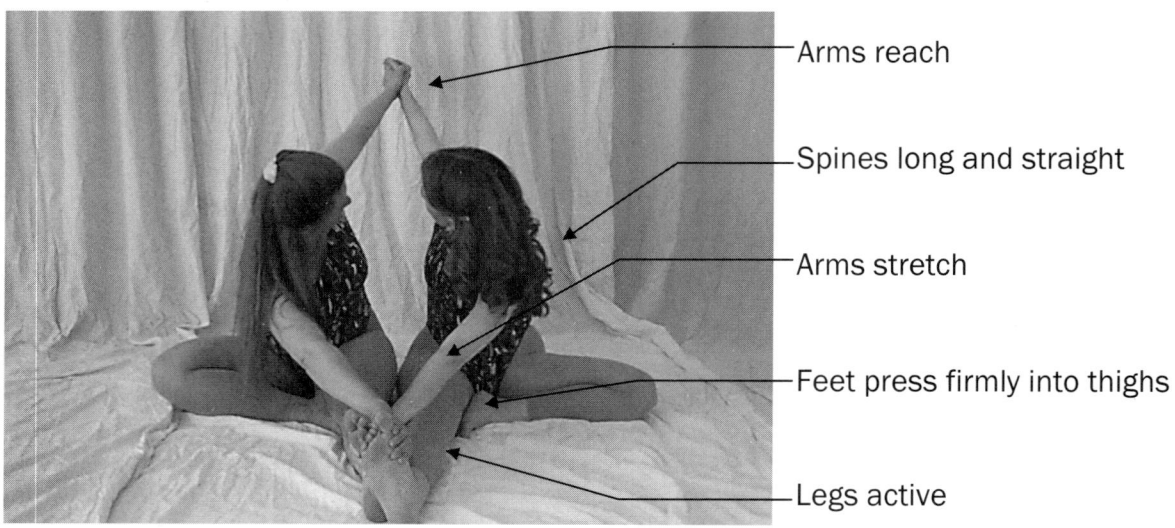

Arms reach

Spines long and straight

Arms stretch

Feet press firmly into thighs

Legs active

Intimacy

Revolving Comet (Parivrtta Janu Sirsasana 4)

All Levels

Instructions
1. Start sitting hip to hip, facing the same direction.
2. Bend the INSIDE legs at the knees and bring the soles of the feet to rest somewhere comfortable on the inside edges of the thighs.
3. Turn towards OUTSIDE legs and use INSIDE arms to reach towards Partner's foot.
4. Clasp OUTSIDE hands and stretch out arms.

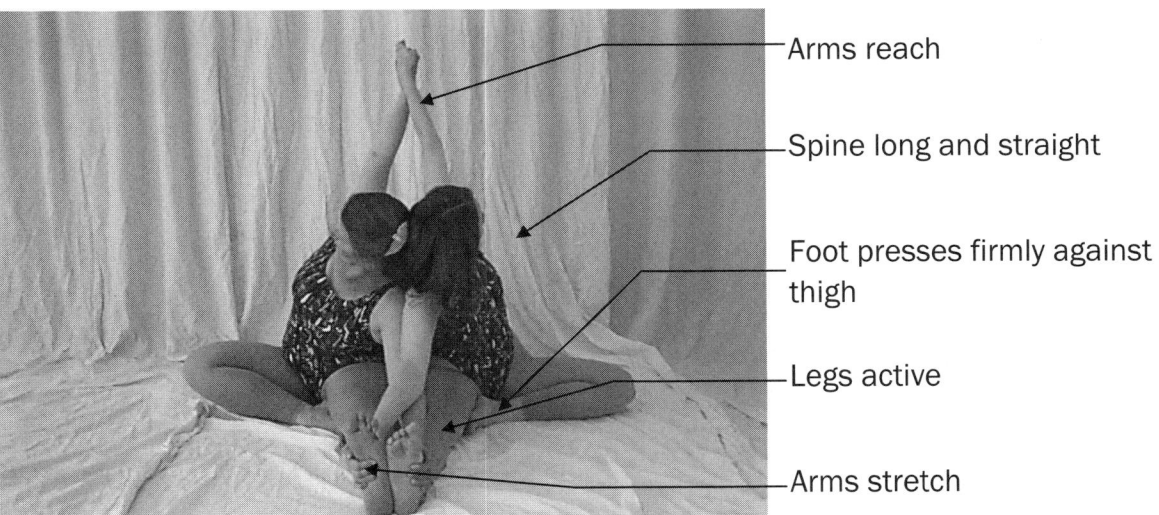

Arms reach

Spine long and straight

Foot presses firmly against thigh

Legs active

Arms stretch

Turning Outward

Spinal Twist (Matsyendrasana)

All Levels

Instructions
1. Start sitting on the floor, face to face and a little more than one leg length apart.
2. Bend LEFT legs at the knee and place the sole of the LEFT foot on the floor as close to the LEFT hip as is comfortable. Place the sole of the RIGHT foot on Partner's LEFT shin.
3. Place RIGHT arms behind backs to support backs.
4. Clasp LEFT forearms, wrists, or hands and twist torsos towards LEFT.

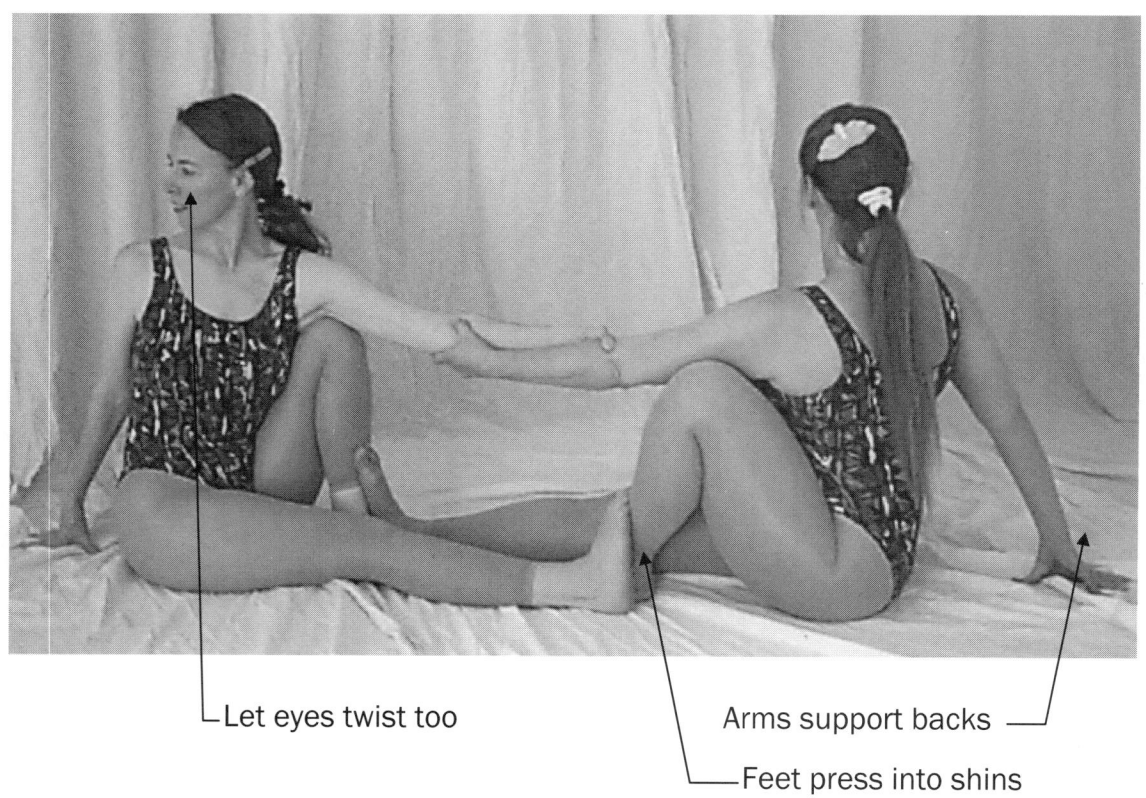

└Let eyes twist too   Arms support backs ─┘

└Feet press into shins

Turning Away from It All

Other Twists

The following is a list of poses where at least one Partner is twisting during the pose or during one part of the pose:

RELAXATION POSES

Press & Release (Apanasana & Standing Squat)

All Levels

Caution - Do not press your Partner's lower legs any farther than is comfortable for them.

Instructions
1. Start with Partner 1 lying in Apanasana as shown.
2. Partner 2 moves in and sits LIGHTLY on Partner 1's lower legs.
3. Partner 1 relaxes completely as Partner 2 slowly rests more and more of their weight on Partner 1.
4. Partner 1 TELLS Partner 2 how much weight to use in the press. After 10 breaths reverse positions.

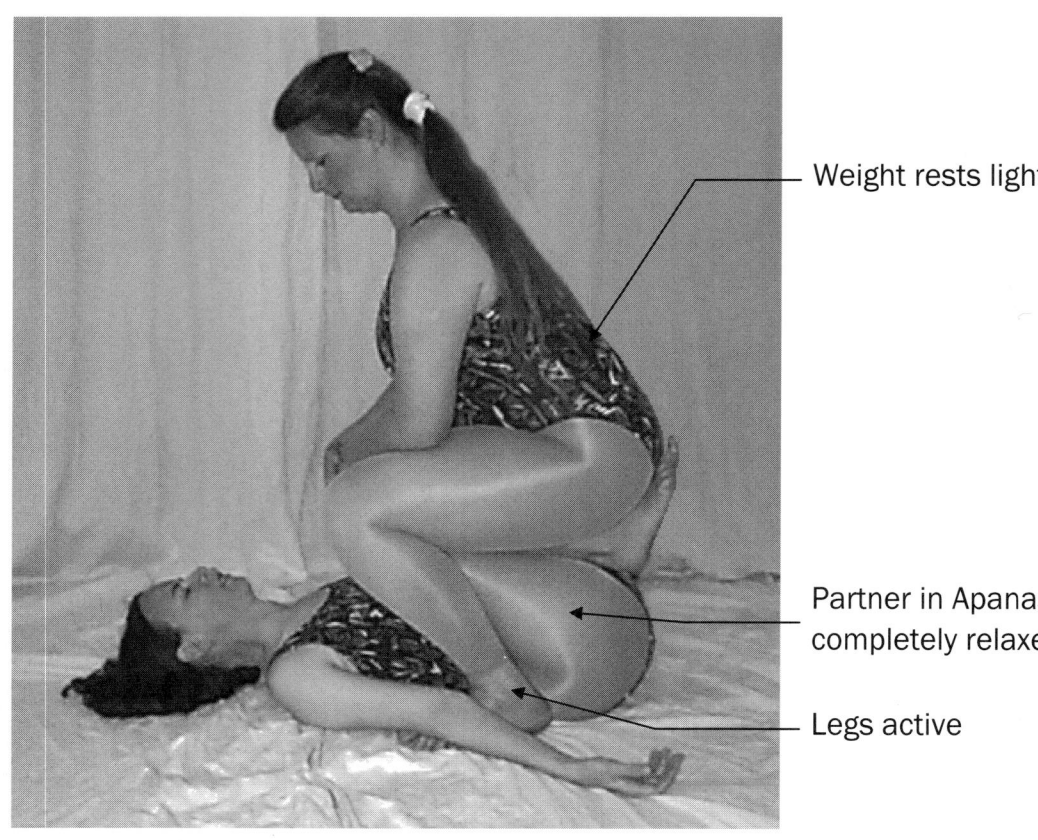

Weight rests lightly on lower Partner

Partner in Apanasana remains completely relaxed

Legs active

With Support Healing Begins

Hip Lift (Savasana & Standing Squat)

All Levels

Instructions
1. Start with Partner 1 on their back with their legs bent at the knees and their feet flat on the floor.
2. Partner 2 moves in facing Partner 1 and straddles their knees.
3. Partner 2 lifts Partner 1's knees until Partner 1's hips and lower back are off the floor and GENTLY shakes Partner 1's hips from side to side and up and down.
4. After 10-12 "shakes" reverse positions.

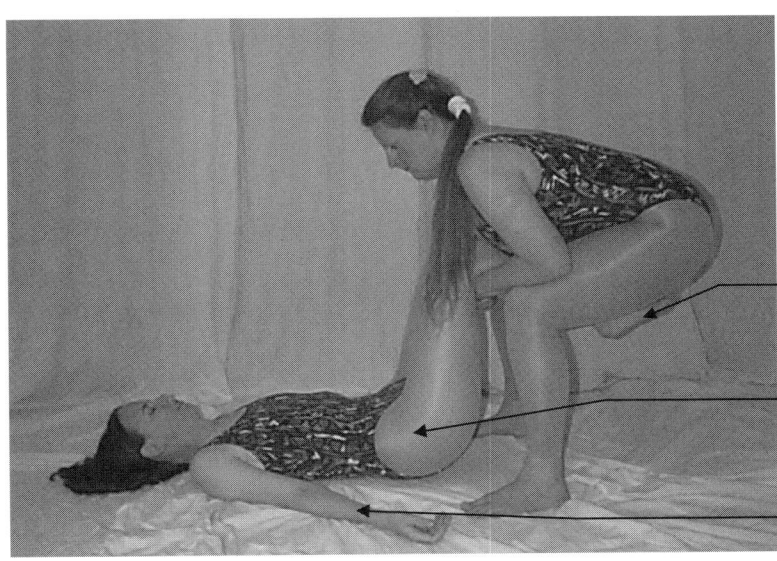

Feet rest on the back of the upper Partner's thighs and hips

Hips and lower back off the floor

Lower Partner completely relaxed

To at Last Give It Up

Torso Lift (Savasana & Tadasana)

All Levels

Instructions
1. Start with Partner 1 on their back with their legs bent at the knees and their feet flat on the floor.
2. Partner 2 moves in facing Partner 1 and straddles their knees.
3. Partner 2 lifts Partner 1's arms until Partner 1's head, shoulders, and mid-back are off the floor and GENTLY shakes Partner 1's upper body from side to side and up and down.
4. After 10-12 "shakes" reverse positions.

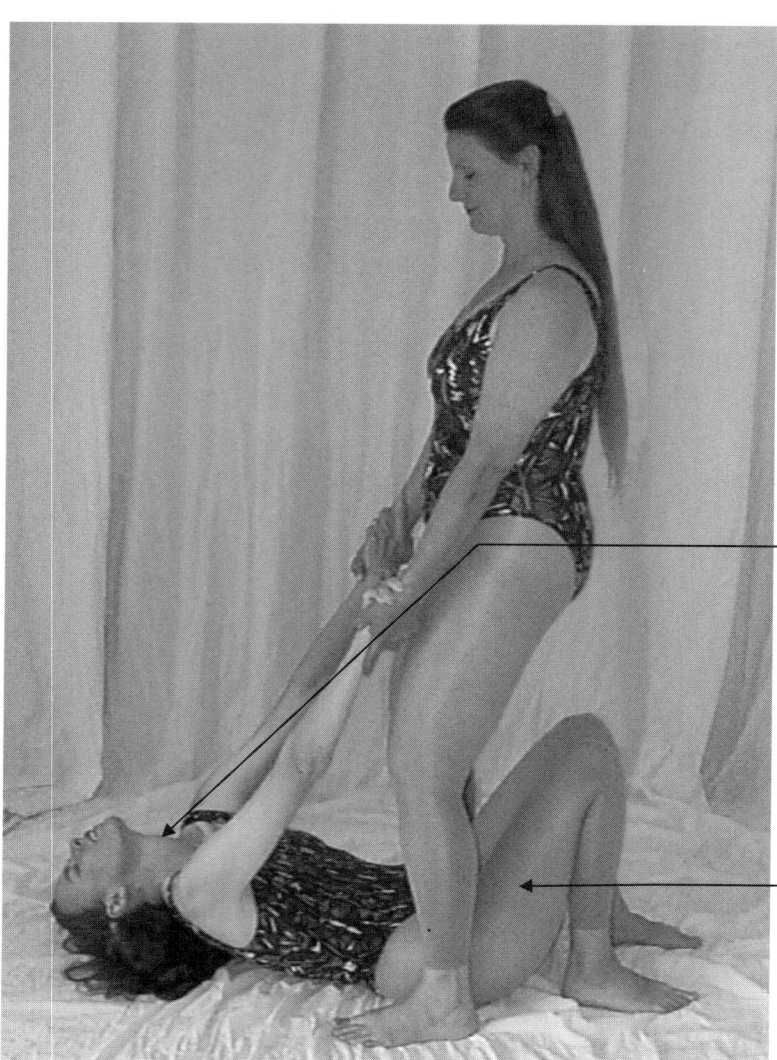

Head, shoulders, and mid-back off the floor

Lower Partner remains completely relaxed

To Give Up all the Rest

Pressed Leaf (Vasisthasana & Balasana)

All Levels

Caution - Do not press your Partner too hard.

Instructions
1. Partner 1 moves into the Child's Pose.
2. Partner 2 places one hand on Partner 1's lumbar vertebra and the other hand on Partner 1's thoracic 7 vertebrae and presses gently, but firmly.
3. Partner 2 massages Partner 1's whole back.

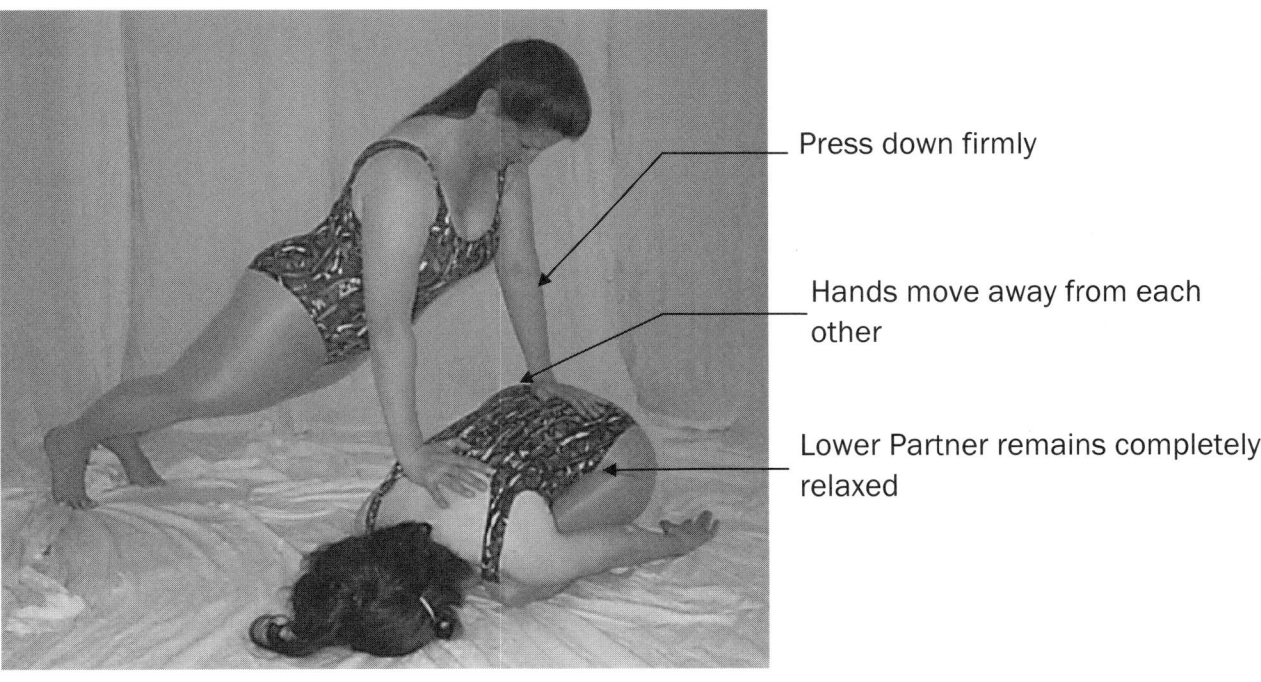

Press down firmly

Hands move away from each other

Lower Partner remains completely relaxed

Making Space in the Chakras

Tao (Setu Bandha Sarvangasana & Sukasana in Paschimottanasana)

Intermediate Level

Instructions
1. Start with Partner 1 sitting in a Forward Bend with their legs in a comfortable cross-legged position.
2. Partner 2 stands with one leg on each side of partner 1's head facing the same direction as Partner 1.
3. Partner 2 sits LIGHTLY on Partner 1's mid-back (NOT LOW-BACK)
4. Partner 2 carefully lies down on Partner 1's back and stretches their arms over their head.

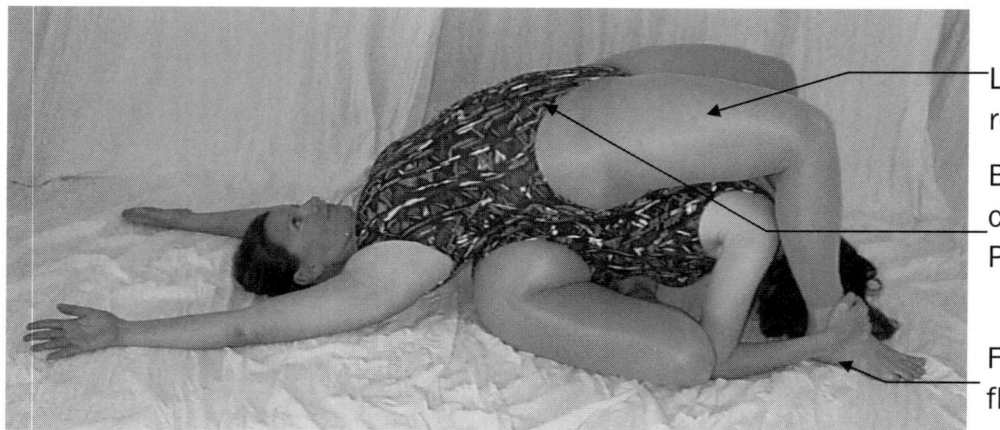

Lower Partner relaxes completely

Body weight centered over lower Partner's hips

Feet pressing into floor

The Yang and the Yin

Pushing the Plough (Halasana)

Intermediate/Advanced Levels

Cautions   - Do not pull/push your Partner any farther than is comfortable for them.
          - You should be thoroughly familiar with the Plough Pose before attempting this pose.

Instructions
1. Start with Partner 1 in the Plough Pose.
2. Partner 2 moves in and sits facing Partner 1's back.
3. Partner 2 grasps Partner 1's wrists and places their feet on Partner 1's mid-back.
4. Partner 2 GENTLY pulls on Partner 1's arms and pushes on Partner 1's back with their feet. Partner 1 remains completely relaxed. After 10 breaths reverse positions.

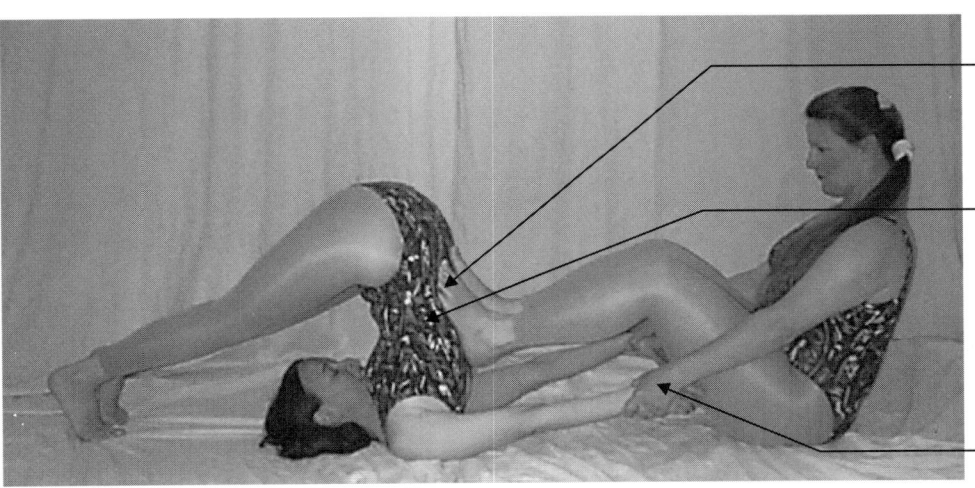

Feet push GENTLY on mid-back and upward

Partner in Plough Pose remains completely relaxed

GENTLY pull on arms

Sowing Seeds for the Soul

Hug Asana (Baddha Konasana)

All Levels

Instructions

1. Start with Partner 1 sitting with the soles of their feet touching and the heels as close to their body as they comfortably can (also called the "Bound Angle Pose").
2. Partner 2 moves in and sits facing Partner 1 with the soles of their feet lightly pressing on the tops of Partner 1's feet.
3. Partners lean forward and place heads on Partners' RIGHT shoulders.
4. Place LEFT arms around Partners' RIGHT torsos and RIGHT arms on Partners' LEFT shoulders. After 5-10 breaths reverse sides.

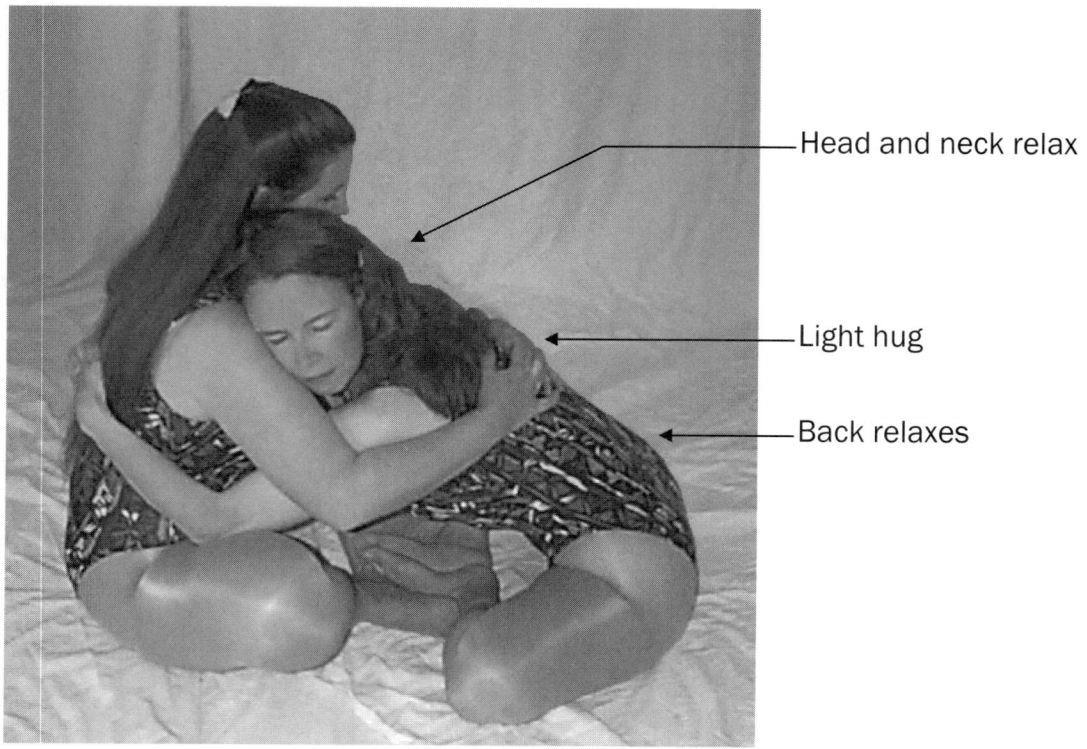

Head and neck relax

Light hug

Back relaxes

Let the Love In

Crown to Crown (Balasana)

All Levels

Instructions

1. Start sitting on heels face to face 4-5' apart (the exact distance will be determined by the height of the Partners).
2. Move into Child's Pose with the crowns of heads touching, arms at sides.

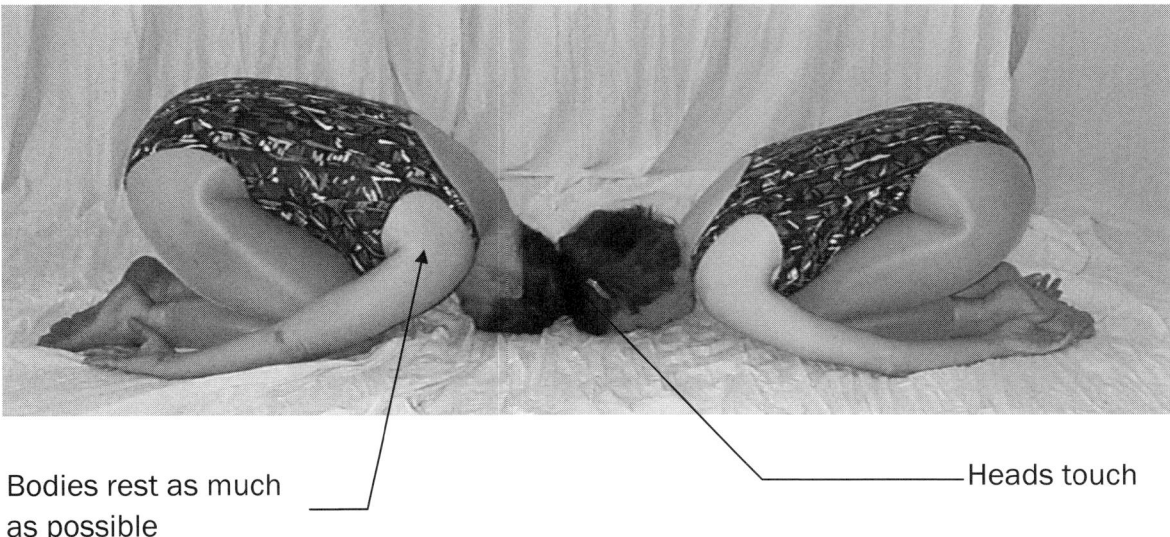

Bodies rest as much as possible

Heads touch

Meeting at the Crown

Heart to Heart (Balasana)

All Levels

Instructions

1. Start sitting on heels face to face 4-5' apart (the exact distance will be determined by the height of both Partners).
2. Move into a mutually agreed upon version of Child's Pose with the crowns of heads touching and hands on Partner's back over heart.

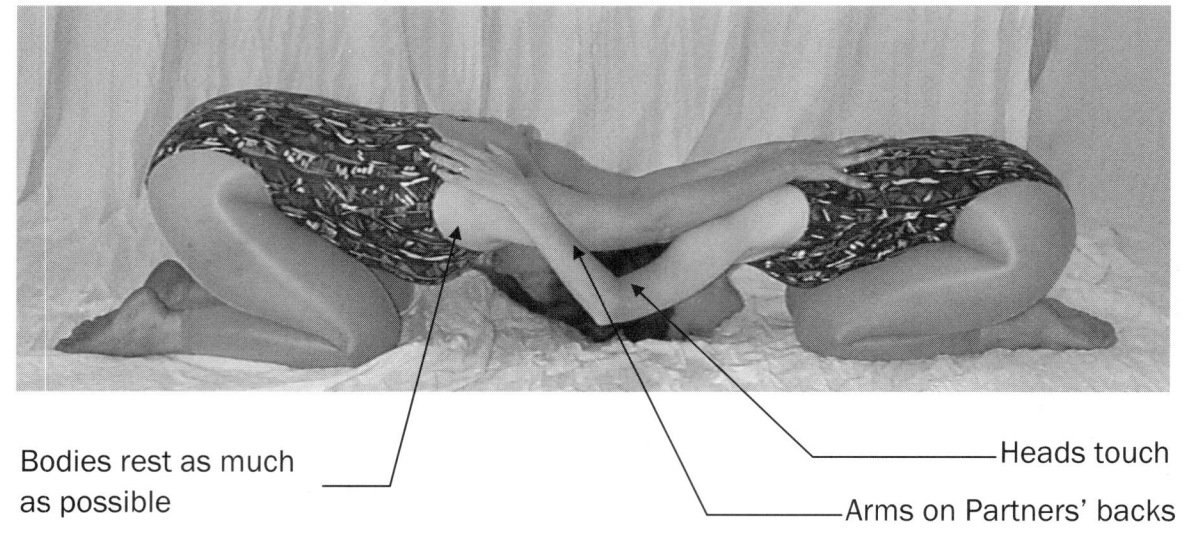

Bodies rest as much as possible

Heads touch

Arms on Partners' backs

Closure

Watchtower (Savasana & A Sitting Pose)

All Levels

Instructions
1. Partner 1 rests on their back on the floor. Their hands can be at their sides or in the Triangle Mudra*.
2. Partner 2 sits in any comfortable position, gazes at Partner 1's diaphragm, and watches Partner 1 breathe.

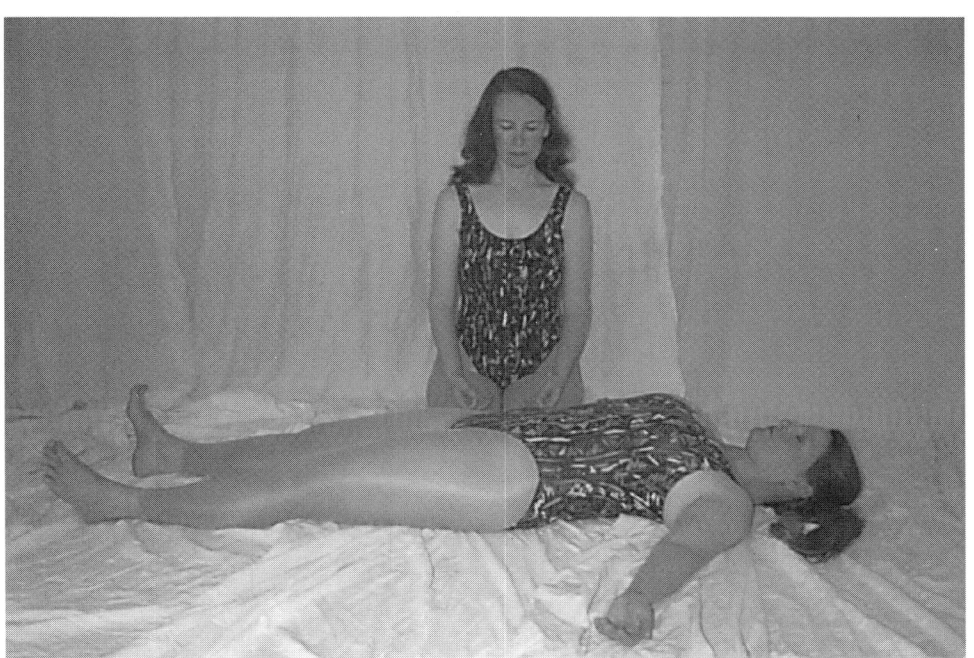

Mandala

* See Table of Contents or Index to locate a picture of this finger position.

Other Relaxation Poses

The following is a list of poses where at least one Partner is relaxing during the pose or during one part of the pose:

Head Garland (Savasana) - page 125
Hip Lift (Savasana & Standing Squat) – page 107
Laugh Chain (Savasana) - page 120
Torso Lift (Savasana & Tadasana) – page 108

GROUP POSES

Breathing Wreath

All Levels

Instructions
1. Arrange group in a circle, facing center, sitting cross-legged, knees touching.
2. Everyone places their RIGHT hand on the back or shoulder of the person sitting to their RIGHT.
3. Everyone places their LEFT hand on the back of the of the person sitting to their LEFT.
4. Breathe together.

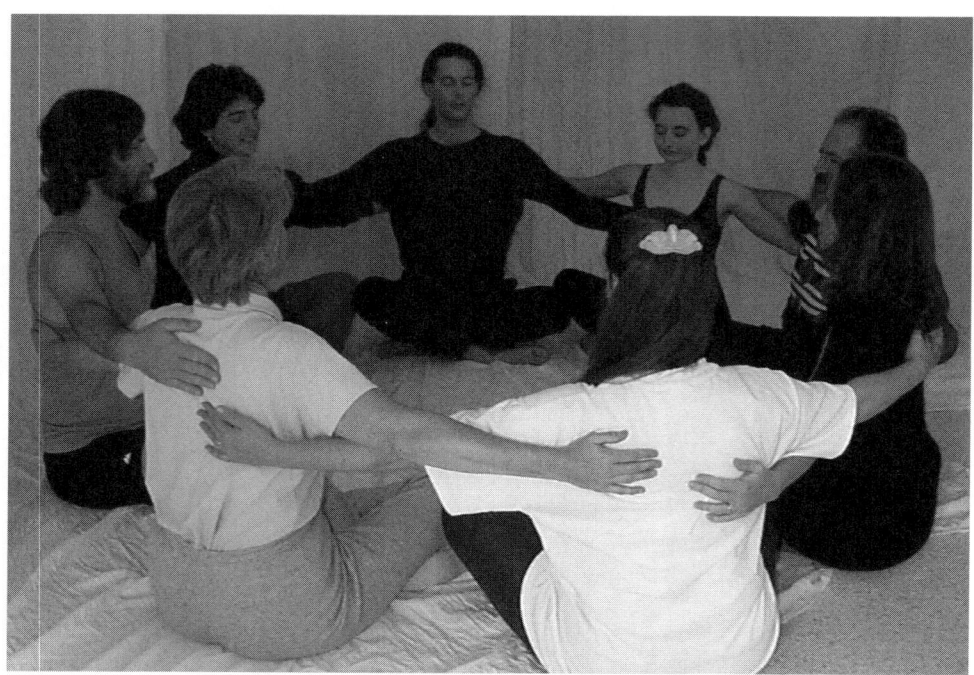

We Are of One Breath.

Kindergarten (Balasana)

All Levels

Instructions
1. Arrange group in a circle, facing center, sitting on heels with 2 hand widths between students.
2. Everyone moves into Child's Pose.

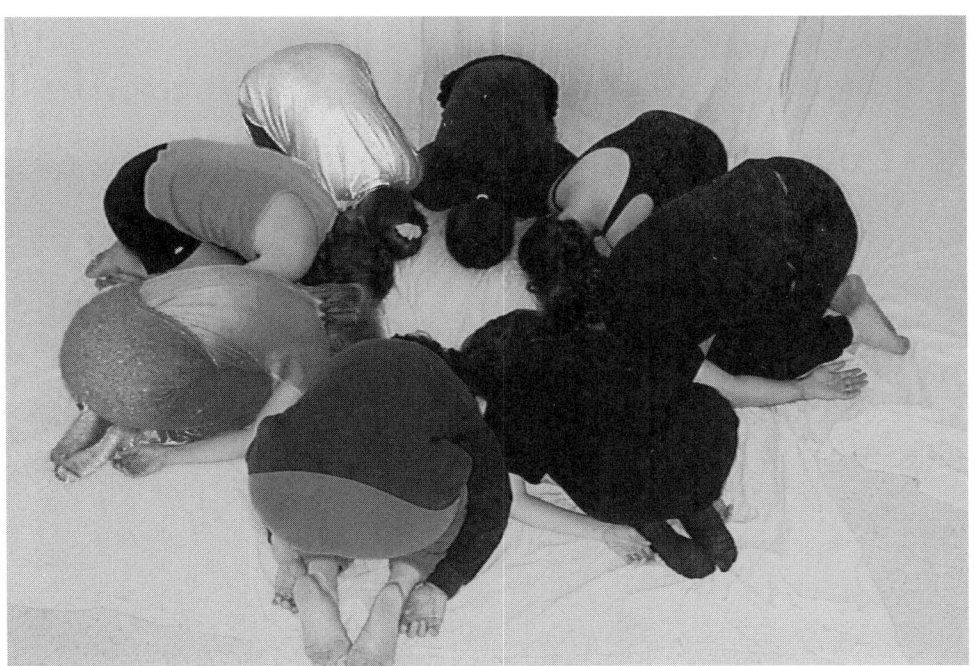

Meeting of the Minds

Laugh Chain (Savasana)

All Levels

Instructions

1. Start with one person lying flat on their back on the floor.
2. The next person lies on the floor at a right angle to the first person and their head on the first person's stomach.
3. Repeat with the remainder of the group zigzagging across the floor until everyone is in position.
4. Tickle one person and watch what happens.

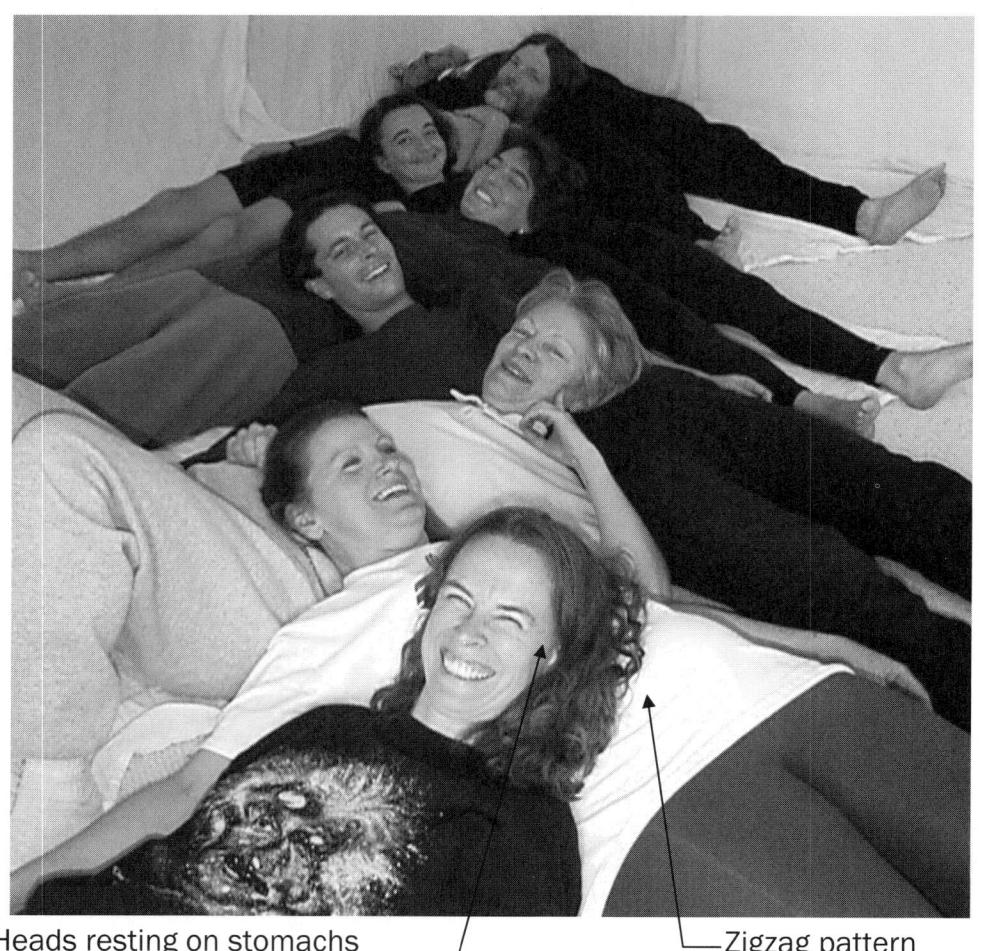

Heads resting on stomachs ——— ———Zigzag pattern

Laughter is Contagious

Hang the Yogi (for 3 or More)

Advanced

Cautions - See individual instructions.

Instructions
1. Start with Partner 1 standing, Partner 2 in Downward Facing Dog Pose behind Partner 1, and Partner 3 standing beside Partner 2 facing him/her.

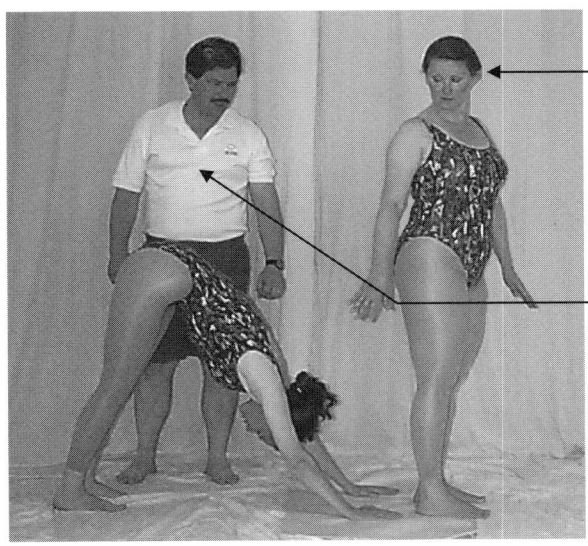

Partner 1's head turned towards Partner 2 before Partner 2 moves into the Handstand

Partner 3 beside Partner 2

2. Partner 3 lifts Partner 2's legs until . . .

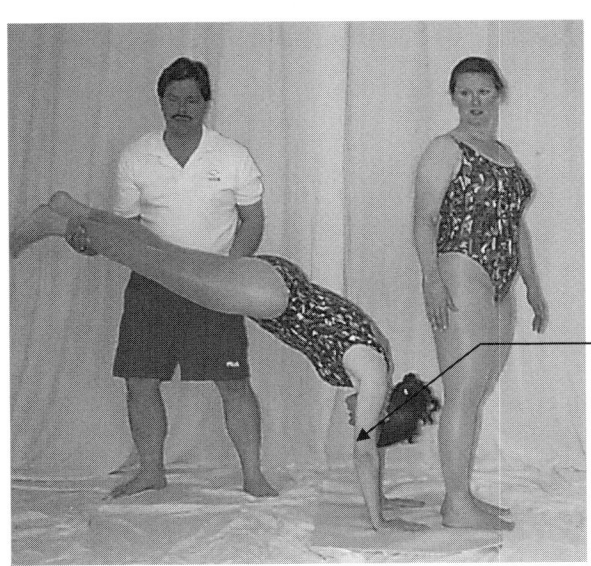

Partner 2 keeps arms straight

3. . . . the backs of Partner 2's legs rest lightly on the back of Partner 1's shoulders. Partner 1 moves into Chair Pose (depth is dependent on Partner 2's height) until the back of Partner 2's knee joints can rest directly on top of Partner 1's shoulders. Partner 1 grips Partner 2's shins, pulls firmly straight outward and stands up straight.

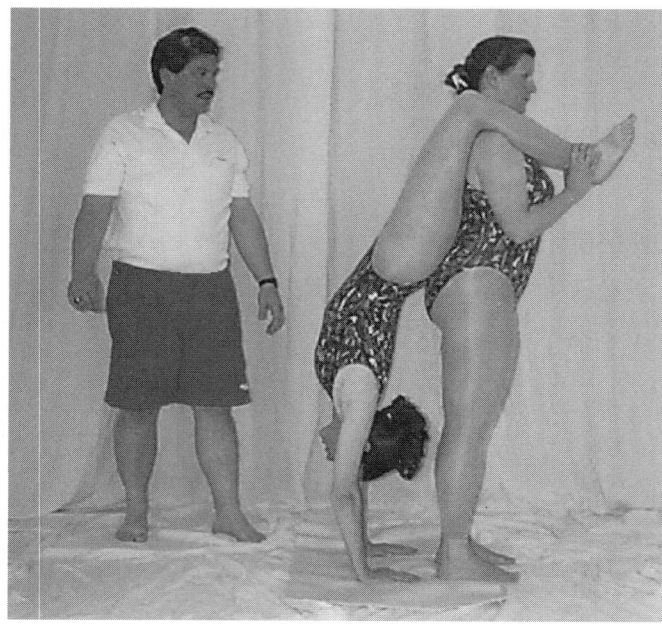

Caution - Do NOT pull lower legs down, pull straight out from shoulders

4. Partner 1 straightens knees and moves into a partial Standing Forward Bend lifting Partner 1 off the floor. Partner 2 grasps Partner 1's ankles/calves. Partners can remain in this part of the pose for up to 1 minute.

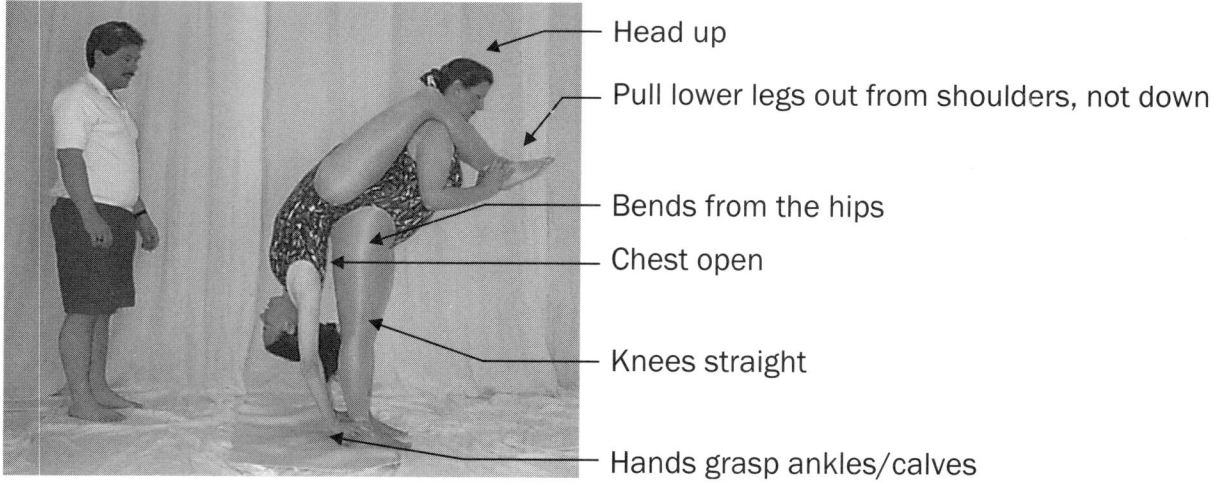

Head up

Pull lower legs out from shoulders, not down

Bends from the hips

Chest open

Knees straight

Hands grasp ankles/calves

5. Partner 2 releases hands and Partner 1 moves farther into the Standing Forward Bend. Partner 1 should keep their head up. Partners can remain in this part of the pose for up to 1 minute.

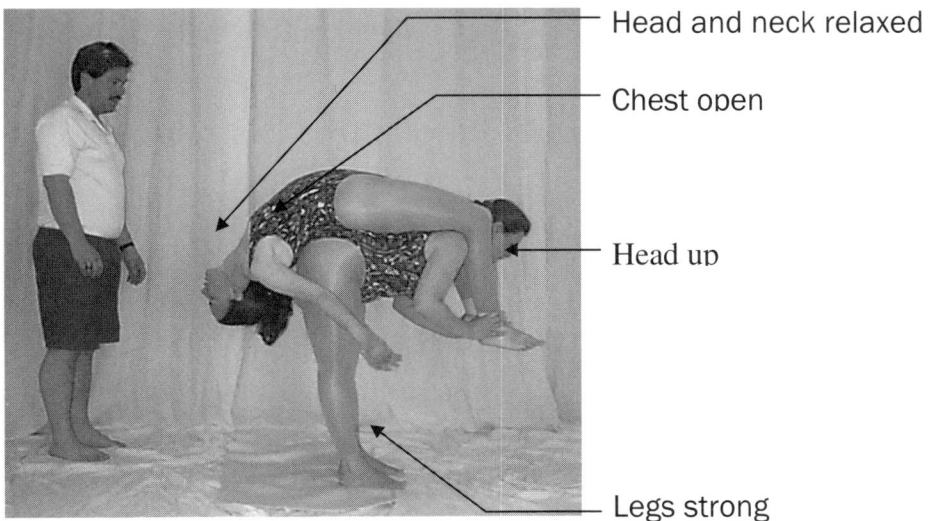

Head and neck relaxed

Chest open

Head up

Legs strong

6. Partner 2 completes Standing Forward Bend and LOWERS their head. Partner 1 moves to standing position.

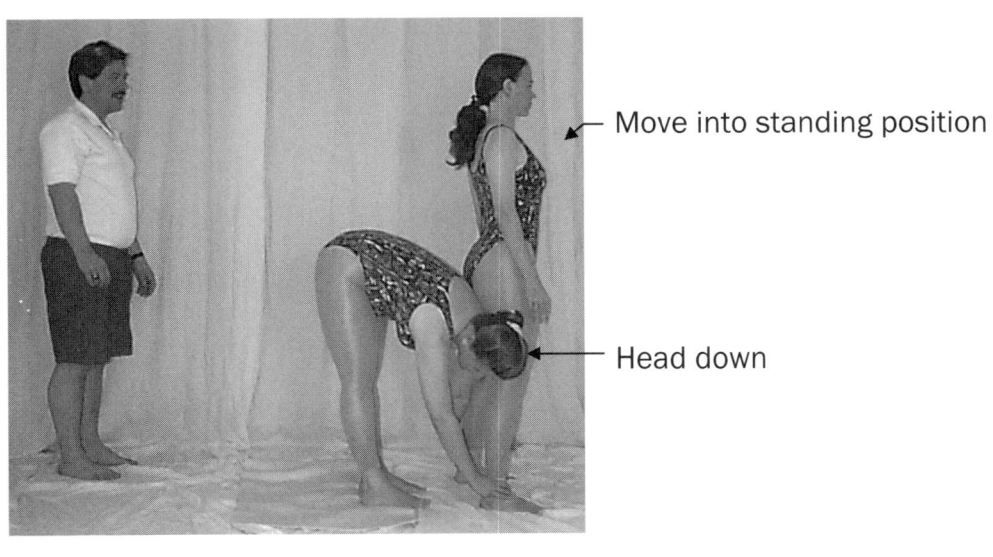

Move into standing position

Head down

Trust

Touching Hearts

All Levels

Instructions
1. Each person in the group picks a partner.
2. Partner 1 takes Partner 2's left hand and places it over their heart. Partner 2 does the same with Partner 1's left hand.
3. The Partners gaze into one another's eyes for a few moments.
4. Change Partners and repeat until everyone has met with everyone else.

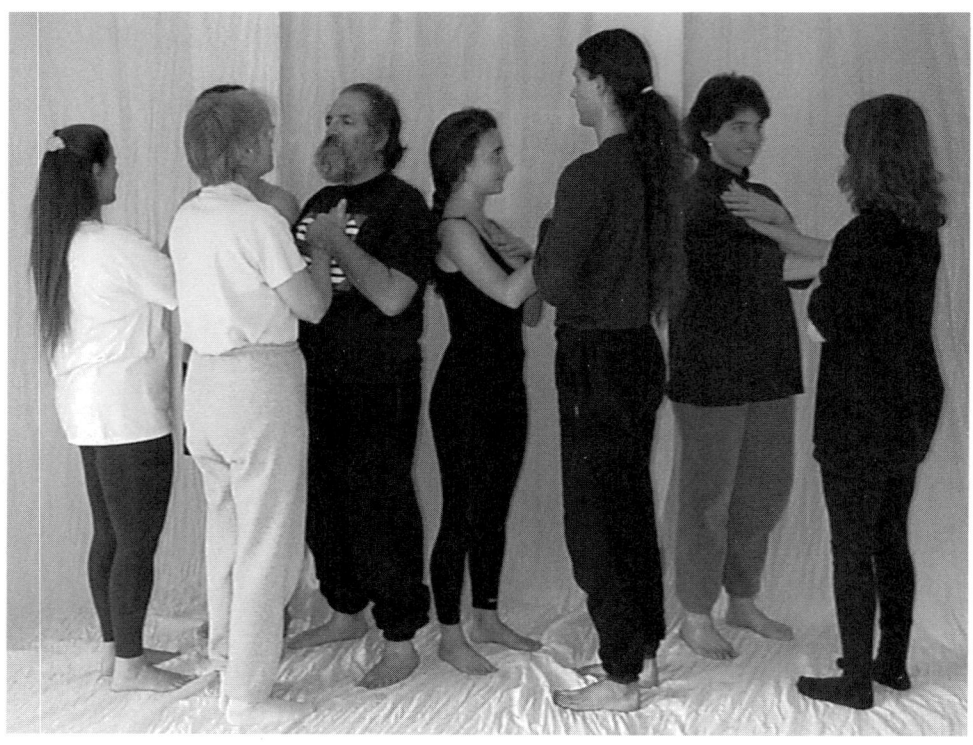

Hands Touching Hearts

Head Garland (Savasana)

All Levels

Instructions
1. All members of the group lie on the floor in a circle with their heads towards the center of the circle and their feet pointing outwards.
2. Everyone moves in towards the center of the circle until shoulders touch.
3. Rest in this position for 5-10 minutes.

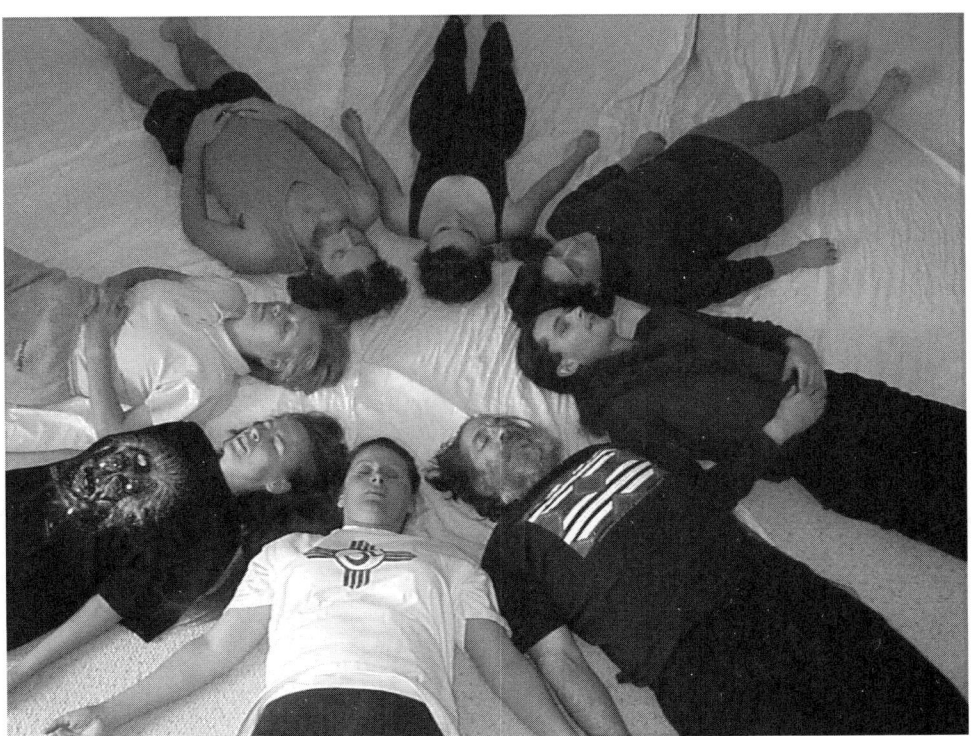

Togetherness

Miscellaneous Poses

Divine or Wisdom Finger Position (Chin or Om Mudra)

All Levels

Instructions

1. Let the tip of each forefinger lightly press into the tip of the thumb on each hand.
2. The amount of pressure between the two fingers should be about the amount necessary to hold a sheet of paper.
3. The other three fingers on each hand can be relaxed or straight but not tense.
4. This mudra helps the breath to flow more evenly. It also help the lungs to fill in a more natural way from bottom to top and use the full capacity of the lungs.

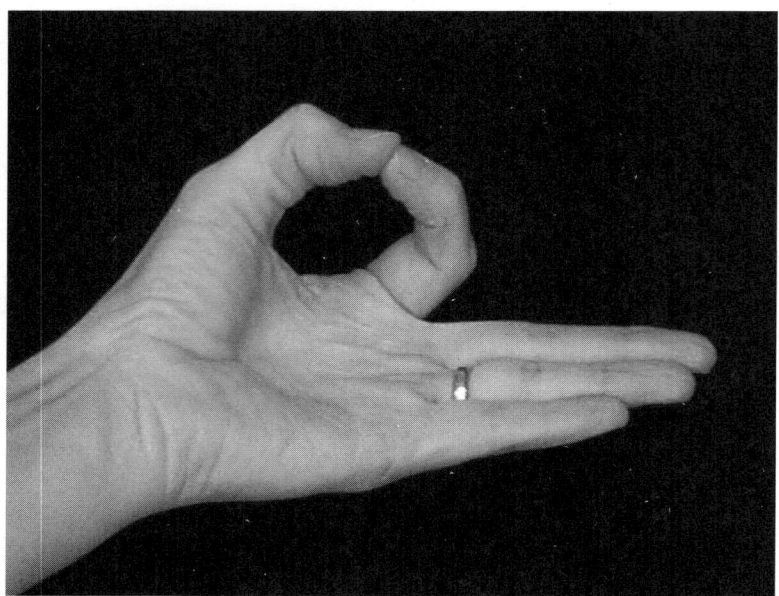

Humility Hand Position (Namaste Mudra)

All Levels

Instructions
1. Place the hands together, palm to palm in front or in back of the upper torso and press in lightly.

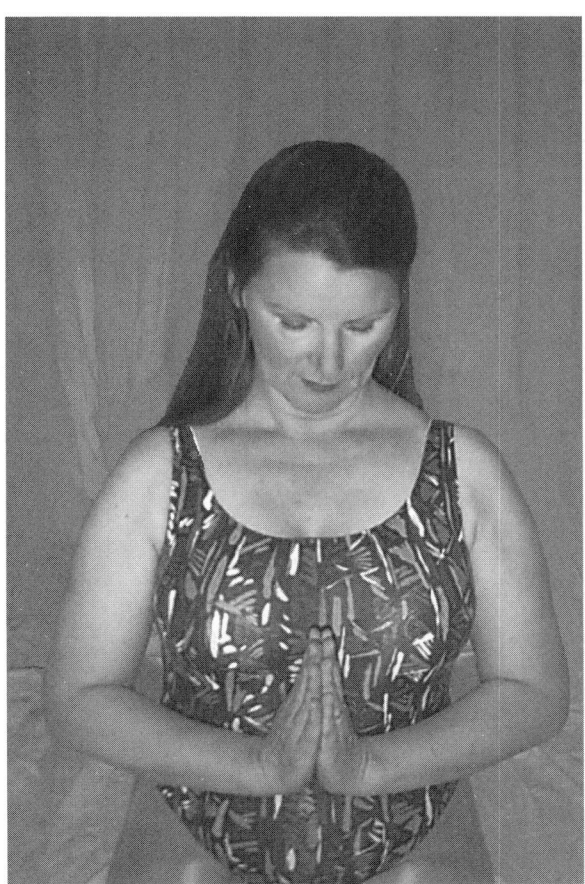 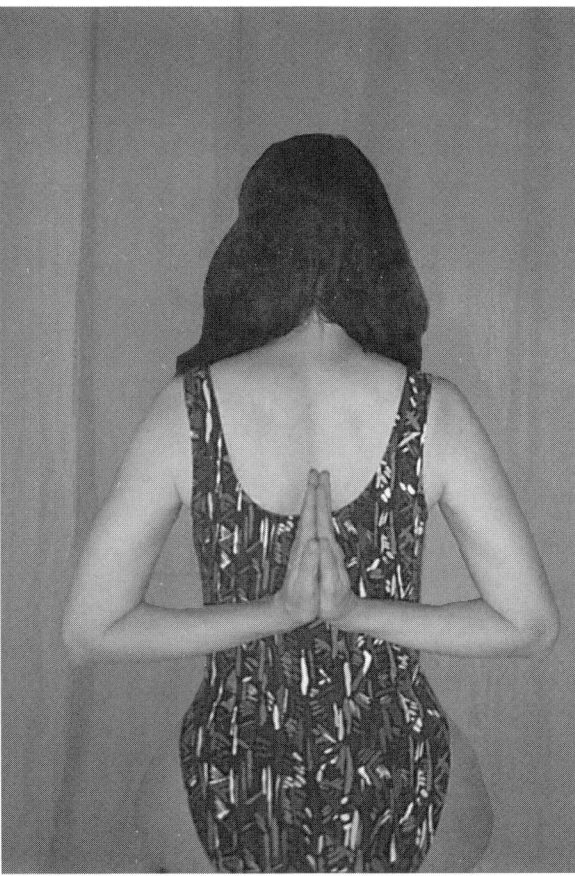

Easy Pose (Siddhasana)

Intermediate/Advanced Levels

Instructions

1. Sit with ankles stacked one on top of the other and bottom heel pressed against perineum.

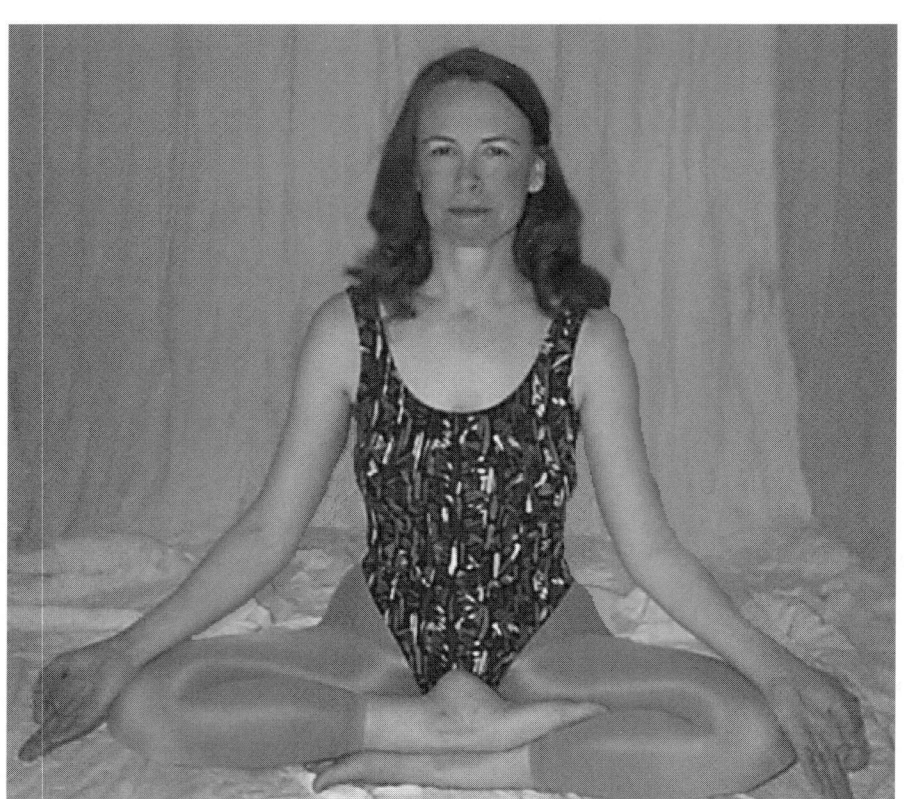

Lotus (Padamasana)

Advanced Level

Caution - If you feel ANY strain in your knees when attempting this pose, DO
    NOT do it.

Instructions
1. Sit with ankles (not feet) on opposite thighs.

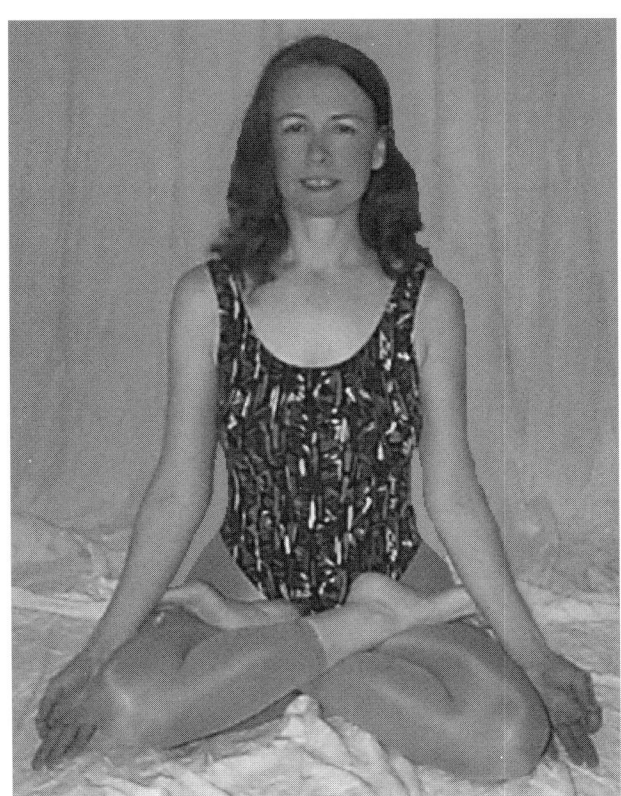

Triangle Mudra

All Levels

Instructions

1. Lie on back and place hands over navel as shown.

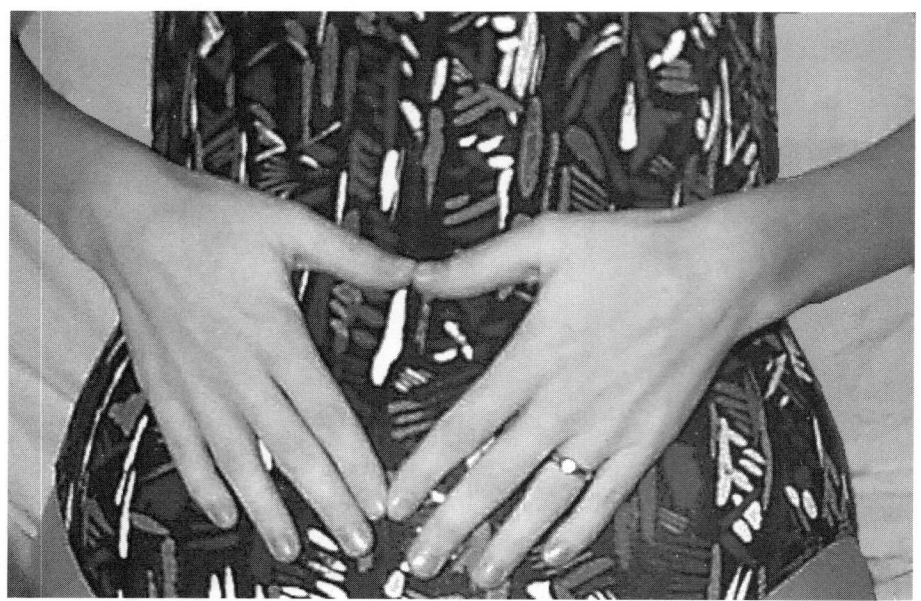

Ujjayi Breath

All Levels

Instructions
1. Assume a comfortable position sitting, lying, or standing.
2. Breathe with the throat slightly closed. This should cause the breath to be audible.

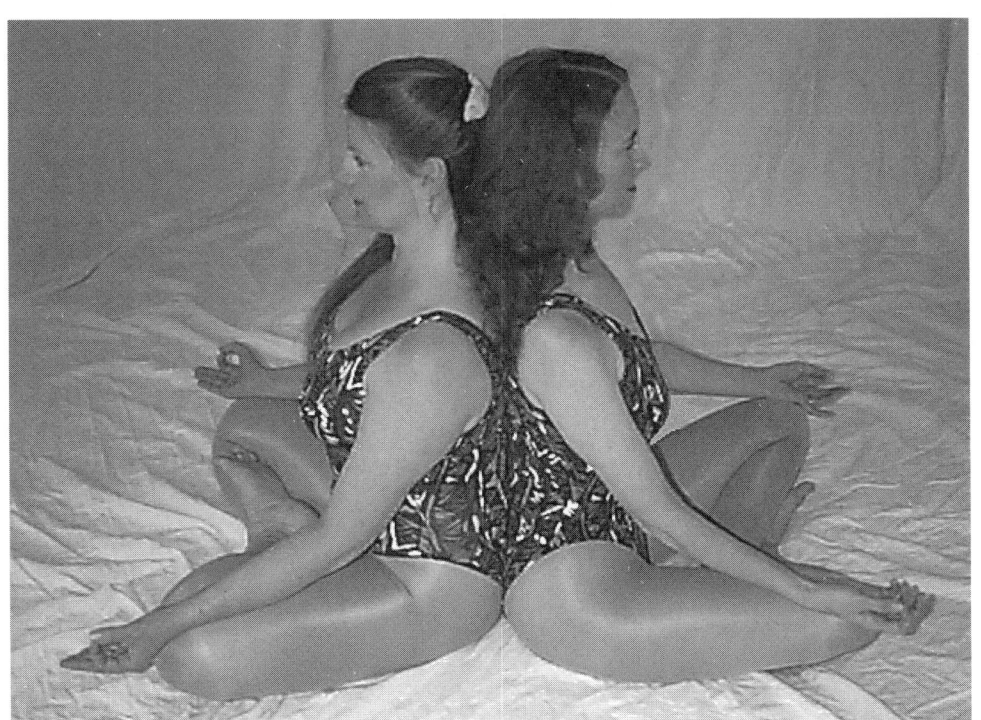

Index

Index, con't.

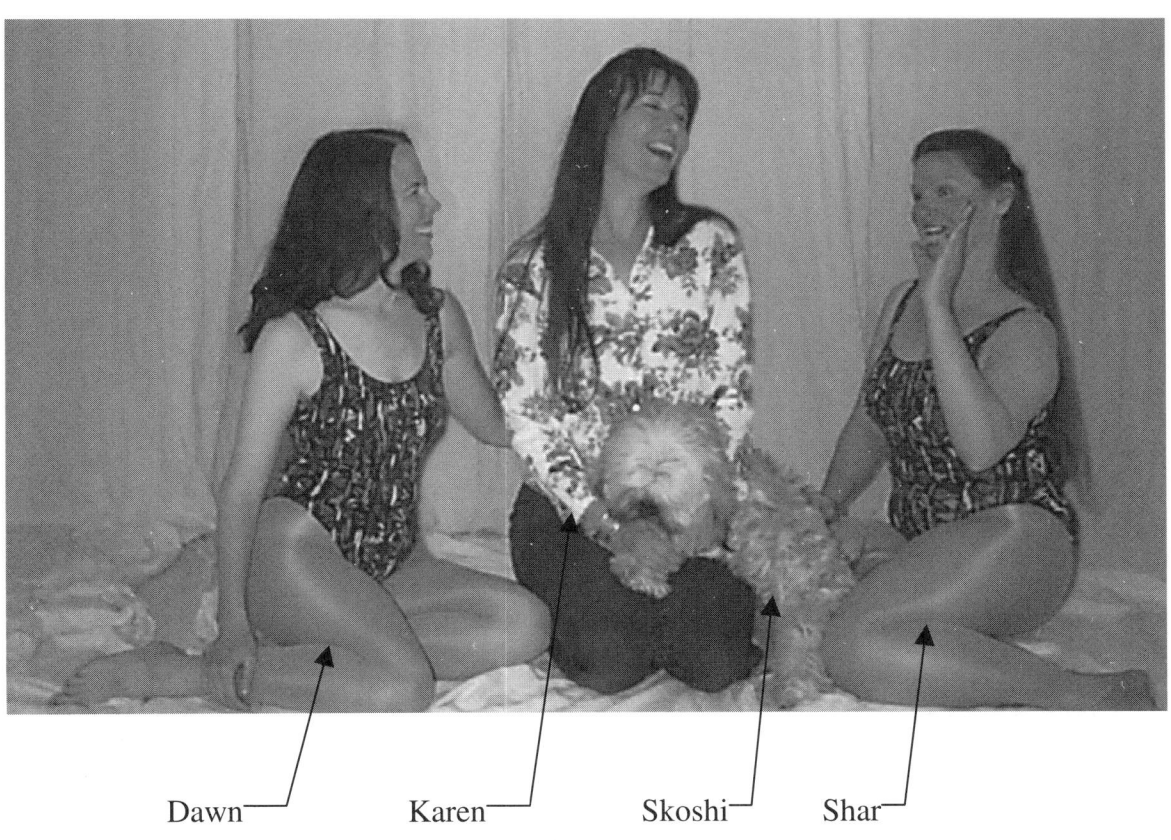

Dawn   Karen   Skoshi   Shar

KRIYA YOGA Publications
Best Selling Titles

BABAJI and the 18 Siddha Kriya Yoga Tradition 4th Edition

By M. Govindan
ISBN 1-895383-00-5
Retail: US $19.95 + $3.00 s/h
C $21.95 +$4.00 s/h

The first authoritative biography of Babaji, the immortal master made famous by Yogananda's **Autobiography of a Yogi**. Babaji lives today near Badrinath, in the upper Himalayan Mountains. His body has not aged since the age of 16, when centuries ago he attained the supreme state of enlightenment and divine transformation. This followed his initiation into the scientific art of Kriya Yoga by two deathless Siddha masters, Agastyar and Boganathar, who belonged to the "18 Siddha Tradition", famous among the Tamil speaking people of south India. This rare account, by a long-time disciple, reveals their little known life stories, ancient culture, and present mission, as well as how their Kriya Yoga can be use to bring about the integration of the material and spiritual dimensions of life. Clear explanations of the psychophysiological effects of Kriya Yoga and guidelines for its practice are given.

-- *"It is the most accurate and comprehensive exposition of the Kriya Yoga tradition and method published in English to date."* – E. Ayyappan, longtime disciple of Babaji.

216 pages, 33 color photos, 4 maps, 100 bibliographic references, and glossary, 6 x 9 inches.

BABAJI's Kriya Hatha Yoga: 18 Postures of Relaxation

By M. Govindan
ISBN 1-895383-03-X
Retail: US $6.00 + $2.00 s/h
C$ 8.50 + $2.35 s/h

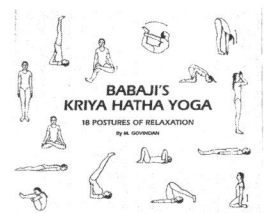

These 18 Hatha yoga postures make an efficient system for rejuvenating the physical body and preparing it for the more subtle phases of Kriya Yoga. Taught in stages and pose/counter pose pairs. Suitable for beginning and experienced students.
30 pages, 6 ½ x 7 inches, softcover.

Kriya Yoga at Badrinath, Himalayas, Video

By M. Govindan
Retail: US $25.00 + $3.50 s/h
C $29.95 + $3.50 s/h
PAL format add US $15

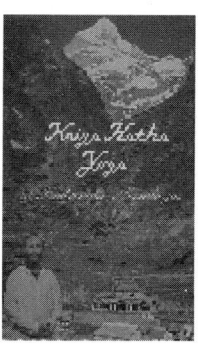

Practice the 18 postures with M. Govindan near Babaji's ashram, amidst breathtaking Himalayan scenery. 58 minutes.

THIRUMANDIRAM:
A CLASIC OF YOGA AND TANTRA

By Siddhar Thirumoolar
Edited by M. Govindan
ISBN 1-895383-02-1
Retail: US $35 per 3-vol set + $6.00 s/h
C $52.00 per 3-vol set + $9.20 s/h

Get connected to the roots of yoga with the first English translation of Thirumoolar's classic masterpiece of yoga, tantra, and Saiva Siddhantha, the gospel of the Tamil Yoga Siddhas. It has inspired the daily life of millions in south India and helped to produce its greatest yogis and saints for the past 2000 years. Written in 3,047 poetic, gem-like verses which go far beyond Patnajali's "Yoga Sutras" in scope and depth, this international edition has been designed to facilitate the reader's understanding with explanatory remarks in the special introductory sections, extensive footnotes, a detailed glossary, index and numerous illustrations. From the most mundane to the most sublime areas of life it provides illuminating guidance and inspiration for Self-realization and Self-transformation.

-- *"The **Thirumandiram** is as important a yoga scripture as the **Bhagavad Gita**, the **Yoga Sutras**, or the voluminous and inspiring **Yoga Vasishtha**. This outstanding text is now available in a fine three-volume edition thanks to Marshall Govindan's labor of love."*—Georg Feuerstein, Ph.D., contributing editor of **Yoga Journal** and the author of the **Yoga-Sutra of Patanjali**, **Sacred Paths**,,and over 20 other books.

828 pages, 6 x 9 inches, in 3 volumes, softcover

How I Became a Disciple of Babaji

By M. Govindan
ISBN 1-895383-04-8
Retail: US $8.00 + $2.00 s/h
C $11.00 + $2.35 s/h

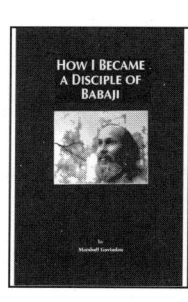

The inspiring story of a young man's quest for God and Self-realization through Babaji's Kriya yoga. From early years of seeking, through ascetic trials in India and Sri Lanka, filled with adventure and difficulties, the author shares a rare story with unusual candor and courage. Rare insights into a little known world.
90 pages, 30 photographs, 6 x 9 inches, softcover.

To Order
VISA: Call toll free in North America: **1-888-252-9642** or
International Orders: **[international code]-800-252-96420**
Check or Money Order, send to:
Kriya Yoga Publications, 196 Mountain Rd., P.O. Box 90,
Eastman, Quebec, Canada J0E 1P0
email: Babaji@Generation.net
web site: http://www.iconn.ca/babaji/

Dr. Emilia Ripoll's Hatha Yoga Tapes for People with Special Needs!
Diabetes – Simple Stress Incontinence – Interstitial Cystitis

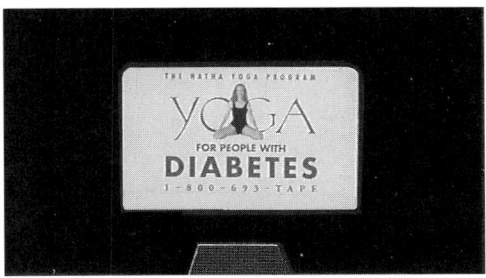

Dr. Emilia Ripoll, MD, a Certified Hatha Yoga Instructor and Licensed Medical Acupuncturist, has designed these Hatha Yoga based exercise videos for people who want special programs geared to their specific needs. These tapes contain exercises based on scientific research and years of practical medical and Hatha Yoga experience.

Produced and directed by Dawn R. Mahowald, CYI, these unique programs are excellent tools for both teachers and students of Hatha Yoga. The directions and movements are presented clearly and concisely in a time tested "watch-then-do" format. Adjustments are given for many poses so people of many different ages and abilities can benefit from the exercises. And, as an added bonus, many poses which stimulate specific acupuncture points for each disorder are included.

DIABETES - $29.95 A 3-part tape with over 30 exercises and variations, suitable for people who's physicians have not limited their physical movements and who are not more than twice their ideal body weight as determined by their physician.

SIMPLE STRESS INCONTINENCE - $24.95 Incontinence is the inability to control the flow and retention of urine. Over half of women and many men over the age of 50 will experience some form of incontinence during their lives. This embarrassing and unpleasant condition can often be controlled with these simple exercises. Can also be suitable for post-partum incontinence.

INTERSTITIAL CYSTITIS - $29.95 This 3-part program includes exercises to help reduce pelvic floor tension, promote stronger, more relaxed lower back muscles, and helps IC sufferers to better relax. Also, uses yoga to stimulate acupuncture points for allergies (a known IC contributor in many patients) as well as those considered important for improved and less painful bladder and kidney function.

TEACHERS - Get all 3 for only $79.95! plus shipping and handling. Perfect for your collection of high quality yoga references.

A Note from Dr. Ripoll - *Our programs are NOT substitutes for a careful, medical evaluation by a qualified physician who deals with your particular disorder. If you currently have symptoms you feel are indicative of a specific disease, but are not certain you have it, seek medical attention from a qualified medical practitioner. Also, ALWAYS check with your doctor before starting any new exercise programs (including ours) and if you have any other limiting physical, mental, or emotional disorders unrelated to your specific physical disorder, you should check with your physician before starting these programs. Please note, our tapes are NOT designed for women who are pregnant.*

To Order
Master Card or VISA: In the USA and Canada call Unique Yoga, Inc. 1-800-693-TAPE (8273)
For orders outside the USA and non-credit card orders send a check or money order to:
Unique Yoga, Inc.
3800 Carlock Dr. #200, Boulder, CO 80303
For shipping and handling add $5.00 for USA and Canadian orders and $10.00 for all others.